Yoga
by the
Numbers

Yoga

by the

Numbers

The Sacred & Symbolic in Yoga Philosophy & Practice

Richard Rosen

SHAMBHALA

Shambhala Publications, Inc.
2129 13th Street
Boulder, Colorado 80302
www.shambhala.com

© 2022 by Richard Rosen

Cover art: MaxyM and 1001holiday/Shutterstock
Cover design: Kate Huber-Parker
Interior design: Kate Huber-Parker

All rights reserved. No part of this book may be reproduced
in any form or by any means, electronic or mechanical, including
photocopying, recording, or by any information storage and retrieval
system, without permission in writing from the publisher.

9 8 7 6 5 4 3 2 1

First Edition
Printed in the United States of America

Shambhala Publications makes every effort
to print on acid-free, recycled paper.
Shambhala Publications is distributed worldwide by
Penguin Random House, Inc., and its subsidiaries.

Library of Congress Cataloging-in-Publication Data
Names: Rosen, Richard (Yoga instructor) author.
Title: Yoga by the numbers: the sacred and symbolic in
yoga philosophy and practice / Richard Rosen
Description: First Edition. | Boulder, Colorado: Shambhala, 2022.
Identifiers: LCCN 2022012482 | ISBN 9781611807387 (trade paperback)
Subjects: LCSH: Symbolism of numbers. | Yoga.
Classification: LCC BF1623.P9 R587 2022 | DDC 181/.45—dc23/eng/20220509
LC record available at https://lccn.loc.gov/2022012482

Dedication to Donald Moyer—

An absolute gentleman,
full of most excellent differences,
of very soft society and great showing.
Hamlet, act 5, scene 2

The world is the veil we spin to hide the void.
Norman O. Brown, "Nothing," *Love's Body*

Contents

Acknowledgments

As always, many thanks to Beth Frankl at Shambhala Publications for her patience and unstinting support. I'd also like to acknowledge my late friend and mentor, Georg Feuerstein, whose *Spirituality by the Numbers* provided the inspiration for this book. As always, whatever is right and good in this book comes from my teachers, all the mistakes are mine alone.

Abbreviations

Advaya Taraka Upanishad	ATU
Atharva Veda	AV
Bhagavad Gita	BG
Brahma Vidya Upanishad	BVU
Brihad Yogi Yajnavalkya Smriti	BYY
Chandogya Upanishad	CU
Darshana Upanishad	DU
Dhyana Bindu Upanishad	DBU
Gheranda Samhita	GS
Goraksha Shatakam	GSh
Guru Gita	GG
Hatha Ratna Avali	HRA
Hatha Yoga Pradipika	HYP
Hatha Tatva Kaumudi	HTK
Katha Upanishad	KU
Kaula Jnana Nirnaya	KJN
Kularnava Tantra	KT

Laghu Yoga Vasishtha	LYV
Mahabharata	MaB
Maha Nirvana Tantra	MNT
Maitri Upanishad	MaiU
Mantra Yoga Samhita	MYS
Mundaka Upanishad	MuU
Rig Veda	RV
Shandilya Upanishad	SU
Shat Cakra Nirupana	SCN
Shiva Samhita	SS
Siddha Siddhanta Paddati	SSP
Tejo Bindu Upanishad	TBU
Varaha Upanishad	VU
Vedanta Sutra	VS
Yoga Cudamani Upanishad	YCU
Yoga Shikha Upanishad	YSU
Yoga Sutra	YS
Yoga Yajnavalkya	YY

Introduction

The old yogis loved numbers, small and big and everything in between. Just as we do today, they used numbers for practical ends: they counted with them, measured, regulated, organized, compared and contrasted, and made connections. But they also used many of those same numbers to tell a story within the story they were numbering, often with an unexpected twist that induced what can only be described as a meditative state.

Take, for example, the yogis' Brahman, the Absolute, from whom the universe emerged, through whom it's sustained, and by whom it will be withdrawn into itself at the end of its life cycle. Imagine, such inconceivable power, and yet one of Brahman's alternate names is *shunya*, which translates into English as "void" and "zero." How is it possible for an entire universe, which as we know today is home to at least two *trillion* galaxies, to the born from, well, nothing?

We'll come back to this soon.

I was well aware—I thought—that there were lots of numbers in the literature, so imagine my surprise—*shock* might not even be too strong a word to describe my reaction—when my research in the old texts unearthed way more numbers than I knew what to do with. Considering the agreed-upon length of the finished version of *Yoga by the Numbers*, it simply wouldn't be possible to include all I'd collected, not to mention those I anticipated were yet to be found. A good portion of them would have to be left out in the cold. I briefly considered changing my title to *Yoga by Some of the Numbers*, but in the end decided against it.

There were two questions I had to answer before writing could proceed. One, among all the numbers stuffing my computer's memory, which should I include and why? And two, under each general number, which specific instances of that number should I include and why?

The first question was fairly easy to answer. I concluded it would make the most sense to focus on the most common numbers distributed throughout the literature—0 through 10—and yes, zero is a number and a rather significant one in the yogis' world.

I also decided on something a bit off the beaten track. Even though number systems have been around since about 4000 BCE, none of them had a zero until it was invented, perhaps in the seventh century CE. There's no argument that the inventor was an Indian, but there's plenty of controversy over who that Indian was. Whoever it was, after more than 4,500 years with no zero, mathematicians and historians agree this invention is one of the crowning achievements of Indian culture, one that enormously benefited all humankind.

I wanted to include the story of zero, but in order to do so, I had to establish a connection between it and Indian spirituality and yoga. Happily, I found several reputable scholars who maintained there was such a connection, and so the first chapter you'll come to will focus on zero.

The second question wasn't quite as easy to answer. A few of the numbers—3, 4, and 5 in particular—are rife with possible subjects. Most of these are mainstream items that would be most relevant and meaningful to modern students. But there were other items that, while not exactly mainstream and probably less relevant, were nonetheless interesting or amusing in their own way. In the end I settled on a combination of both, leaning a little more toward the mainstream.

Since my highest numbered chapter is 11, I also had to find a way to include significant higher numbers. A few—such as 16, 18, 84, and that most yogic of yoga numbers, though no one's quite sure why, 108—definitely couldn't be ignored. So when the story calls for it, each of these numbers will be discussed in a subsection titled Behind the Numbers. This same heading will also indicate a short detour from the subject at hand to inject some background information. You'll also find here and there a short illustrative story, such as the Origin of Hatha Yoga, or simple practice that somehow puts into action something discussed in the book.

▸ ▸ BEHIND THE NUMBERS

Number and Numeral

> *Number*, from Latin *numerus*, from √*nam*, "to allot, count out, portion out."
>
> Etymology of *number*

Before we begin, we should first note the difference between a *number* and a *numeral*. The former is something we've counted or measured that we hold in our mind; the latter is that number in our mind that's been written down in standard symbols. For example, I've counted the number of fingers and toes on my body, which comes to 20. When I write this number down, the two followed by zero, *2-0*, is a numeral. For the sake of simplicity, we'll call both a number and a numeral a *number*.

▸ ▸ BEHIND THE NUMBERS

Sanskrit Spelling and Pronunciation

Practically all the traditional texts I consulted for this book were originally written in Sanskrit. Sanskrit does something formally with its spelling that we English speakers sort of do with our everyday speech. Say to yourself the words, "Come on." Reading them, you might be on your best behavior and pronounce them clearly as two separate words. But usually we would tend to blend the words together when speaking and say something more like, "C'mon."

Sanskrit blends words too—but formally in its spelling. The practice is called a junction (*sandhya*), which you may be familiar with in the names of common *asanas*. Take *pashcimottanasana*. It consists of three words, *pashcima*, *uttana*, and *asana*. We won't concern ourselves with *asana*, but to blend the first two words then, the final *a* of *pashcima* and the initial *u* of *uttana*, according to the rules of sandhya, blend to become an *o*, which you see between the *m* and the first *t* in the full word.

The result of these sandhyas in the Sanskrit texts arelonglinesof-separatewords blended together, which for non-Sanskritists can make reading difficult. To help you with that—and in this I'm assuming that Sanskrit isn't your first or even second language—I've committed a terrible Sanskrit sin and separated blended words into their individual components. So instead of the title *Hatharatnavali*, for example, you'll see *Hatha Ratna Avali*. Hard-nosed Sanskritists will be horrified, and to them, my sincerest apologies.

You should also be aware that what's usually referred to as the Sanskrit alphabet is something of a misnomer. Sanskrit vowels are single letters, like all of the letters in our Roman alphabet. But Sanskrit consonants each carry an innate, unwritten *a*, pronounced "uh." So the Roman *k* is pronounced "kay," but the same character in Sanskrit is pronounced "kuh." Since the characters used to write Sanskrit are a combination of an "alphabet" and a "syllabary," what's usually called the Sanskrit alphabet is technically what's known as an alpha-syllabary.

The characters of the alpha-syllabary are collectively called *nagari*, which means something like "city," suggesting these characters were invented by sophisticated urban dwellers. Sometime along the way, the word *deva*, "god," was attached to *nagari*. This was meant to further suggest the "city" was located in a heaven realm and populated by the gods, making *devanagari* a sacred language. My innate skepticism gets the best of me here, so we'll continue to refer to the alpha-syllabary as simply nagari.

There are two more things I should mention about my Sanskrit transliteration. First, the nagari *c* is pronounced like the *ch* in "church." To help non-Sanskritists with pronunciation then, it's quite common for transliterations to add an *h* after a *c*, so that a word properly spelled *cakra* is modified to *chakra*. I've left the *c*'s well enough alone, so please remember how they're pronounced; for example, *cakra* is pronounced CHUCK-ruh.

Second, in nagari there's something called an *r*-vowel. I won't go into the details, but it's transliterated as an *r* with an underdot. When it's used in a word, it's not followed by a vowel, and so you'll see a word like *vrksha*, "tree." To help non-Sanskritists with pronunciation here, it's quite common for transliterations to add an *i* after a *r*, so that the example word would be spelled *vriksha*. This is what I've done for all the r-vowels.

◂ ◂

1

ZERO (THE VOID) BY THE NUMBERS

The Zero-concept is not only a mathematical discovery, but was originally conceived as a symbol of *Brahman* and *Nirvanam*. Zero is not a single cipher, positive or negative (growth and decay) but the unifying point of indifference and the matrix of the All and the None. . . . It is *shunya*, the primary or final reservoir of all single shapes and numbers.

Betty Heimann, *Facets of Indian Thought*

What do you think about when you think about zero? Nothing, right? Something that's "zero" has "no measurable value" and an "absence of quantity." When we say that a person is a "zero," we're not being very kind, we're suggesting that they have "no influence or importance," that they are a "nonentity." Some people aren't even sure zero is a number; they think it's merely a placeholder of no particular consequence.

The invention of zero perhaps 1,400 years ago was a breakthrough of major consequence for the entire world, and we have the Indians to thank for that. It wasn't just mathematics affected by this number, as we see in the quote from Professor Heimann. The sages took zero a step farther and made it the universal "matrix of the All and the None." They also discovered this same empty fullness at the core of our being.

What would we do if our number system didn't have a zero? Do you think it's not possible not to have a zero? Let's look back more than 5,000 years ago to Sumer, located in Mesopotamia between the Tigris and Euphrates Rivers and home to one of the world's earliest civilizations. The Sumerians are remembered for a variety of firsts or near-firsts: they were at the forefront of developing astronomy, a legal system, animal husbandry (cattle and sheep), and agriculture. Around 3400 BCE, they also invented the first number system. Unlike our base 10 number system—with its 10 numbers (including zero)—the Sumerian system was sexagesimal, that is, base 60. Here we have the origin of our 60-second minute, our 60-minute hour, and a circle with 360 degrees. What may seem odd to us is that although this system had 59 numbers, it had no zero.

Why? In the times before people lived in large, settled communities, they roamed about in small, tight-knit groups. Of necessity, possessions were few, so counting things was unnecessary. It's been speculated that numbers were originally invented solely for the practical purpose of keeping track of an ever-increasing number of people, livestock, and resources in market transactions as the civilization was established, expanded, and prospered. Counting things then made sense: "I'll trade you five of these for eight of those"—someone could hold five things and see the eight things he wanted. But we can't barter nothing for another nothing, nor would we barter something for nothing. Zero then seemed to have no practical value and so went un-invented.

But zerolessness presented a problem. When writing a number like 108 (and here I'm using modern numbers for the purpose of this illustration; the Sumerian numbers naturally were much different), the Sumerians left a blank space where the zero would have been had they invented one. So their 108 was written like this: 1_8, with an underline to indicate the blank space. As you can see, as long as we all know the blank space stands for zero and it's flanked and so contained directly on either side by numbers, there isn't much confusion. But what happens when the blank or blanks come at the end of a number? How did the Sumerians tell the difference between 3 and 3_ (30) and 3_ _ (300)? Apparently, or maybe hopefully, the number's context hinted at the correct choice.

This hit-and-miss numbering isn't, as you can imagine, the best way to keep track of a larger amount of people or cows or to engage in trade. What the Sumerians needed was a placeholder, a mark positioned to the right of at least one digit other than zero, that itself stands for zero. They exited the scene without ever figuring that out. Eventually, sometime between 400 and 300 BCE, the Babylonians, who followed the Sumerians and inherited their number system, invented a mark—a pair of parallel wedges—that served as that placeholder. This simple solution helped clear up the possible confusion caused by the blank spaces, but it wasn't yet a number. That would take another 700 to 800 years, maybe more.

This raises a question about zero as a number. We in the West generally think 0 stands for nothing, and nothing more. If this is so, then how can zero be a number? If a number is something we count with, a "mathematical unit used to express an amount, quantity, etc.," it seems fair to ask, what can we count with nothing? Isn't zero just a placeholder used with actual numbers to indicate the absence of a number, as it was with the Babylonians?

Modern mathematicians unequivocally accept 0 as a number. To put it as simply as possible, 0 isn't nothing; it's the number that stands for nothing, positioned on the number scale between -1 and +1. Like every other number, we can add, subtract, and multiply with 0, though it was proven in the early eighteenth century that, unlike every other number, dividing by 0 is impossible. So despite any lingering doubts, we must grudgingly accept 0 as a number, even though, like Shakespeare's idiot's tale, it "signifies nothing."

The mathematicians and number historians generally agree that zero was invented in ancient India, though exactly by whom, how, and when is still a matter of heated debate. There are, as far as I could discover, four candidates for the title "inventor of zero."

The most favored of the four among those in the know is a mathematician-astronomer by the name of Brahmagupta. In a manuscript titled the *Brahma Sphuta Siddhanta* and dated around 628 CE, he laid out extensive rules for computing with zero, represented by a solid dot.

Then there's the unknown author (or authors) of what's called the Bakhshali manuscript, which is essentially an arithmetic primer for merchants, the earliest sections of which were written sometime in the third century CE. Also in the running is a Jain monk named Sarvanandin, who authored a book on cosmology in 458. And finally we have Aryabhata, another mathematician-astronomer, who wrote a major work on mathematics and astronomy around the year 500, when he was 23 years old. His case as the inventor of zero is championed by French scholar Georges Ifrah. Ifrah insists that, although he didn't use the symbol, Aryabhata's work with square and cubic roots would have been impossible without a knowledge of zero.

► ► BEHIND THE NUMBERS

Sanskrit Words for Zero (shunya, kha, bindu)

Sanskrit, the predominant language of traditional yoga, has at least three words for zero. The most common of these, *shunya*, has a host of meanings: it's "empty, void, hollow; barren, desolate, deserted," but also means "space, heaven, atmosphere." It's "vacant (as a look or stare), absentminded, it has no certain object or aim," so it's "distracted." It possesses nothing and is wholly destitute. Alone or solitary, it has no friends or companions. It's free from wants and lacks, even existence itself. A person who is shunya is a "vacuity, a nonentity"—we might unkindly call them a "zero"—as well as "vain, idle, unreal, nonsensical, and guileless, innocent, indifferent, their actions are void of results, ineffectual." All of these words attest to the utter emptiness of *shunya*.

A second zero word is *kha*. Like *shunya*, *kha* is "hollow, an empty space," as well as "sky" and "heaven." It's also the hole in the nave of a wheel through which the axle runs. When that hole is accurately centered in the wheel so the wheel rolls smoothly along the road, we have a "good space," *sukha* (*su* is Sanskrit for "good, easy, right"). But when the hole is off center, we have a "bad space," *duhkha* (*dus* is Sanskrit for "bad"; when *dus* is combined with *kha*, the *s* becomes an *h*), and a bumpy ride. In the yoga lexicon, *duhkha* means "pain, sorrow, trouble, difficulty; it is difficult to or to be; to be sad or uneasy."

A third word for zero, less common than the first two, is *bindu*, a "detached particle, drop, globule, dot, spot." See that little dot after the word "spot" that ends the previous sentence? We call it a "period," but a yogi might call it a *bindu*.

◂ ◂

I should add that while I couldn't find any criticism specifically of this position, it was pretty easy to discover a host of mathematicians who are extremely critical of Ifrah's writings. Since I'm not a mathematician, I have no way of judging who's "right" here and whether or not Ifrah deserves the professional disrespect. I won't quote directly from Ifrah's detractors, except to say they totally dismissed his work. However, in his defense, I found the sections on India in his 600-page tome, *The Universal History of Numbers* (1981), fascinating reading.

If we objectively weigh the pros and cons for all four candidates, we'd have to conclude the inventor of zero, like beauty, is in the eyes of the beholder, that one person's placeholder is another's number. While there's no doubt Brahmagupta used zero as a number and understood it well—though he did try to divide by zero, which is impossible—there's no incontrovertible proof he invented it. As for Aryabhata, while Ifrah's backing keeps him in the running, considering this author's reputation among his colleagues it seems prudent to take it with a grain of *le sel*. It's also possible that none of the four was the inventor and the inventor's name has slipped between the cracks of history and been lost forever, or zero wasn't invented by any one individual and instead the concept was refined over time as it passed through the hands of two or more mathematicians.

Since zero nowadays is a common presence in our lives, it's difficult for us to comprehend the enormous impact the invention of that number had on human culture. Scholar Ifrah notes that along with a pair of other Indian innovations—numerical notation (e.g., 1, 2, 3, 4, etc.) and place value—the zero enabled the "democratization" of calculation. For thousands of years this field had only been accessible to the privileged few (professional mathematicians). These discoveries made the domain of arithmetic accessible to anyone."[1] For good measure, zero also allowed the use of negative numbers and decimal fractions and played an important role in the development of algebra and calculus. (And we all know how valuable algebra and calculus have been in our lives since learning them in high school.) Finally, without zero, there might be no binary number system—the zeros and ones without which it would be impossible for computers to function. If that were so, right now I'd be pecking away at my prehistoric Underwood, my gallon jug of white-out at my elbow.

You may find all of this interesting, but at the same time wonder: *What has this got to do with yoga and numbers?* There's speculation that, among all the ancient cultures, the number zero could only have emerged in India. Why? Because the Indians knew something about nothing that drew them to it, unlike their neighbors, who very naturally feared and shied away nothingness. In fact, through their practices, the yogis actively sought to empty their consciousness of any and all ideation and become nothing themselves, which, paradoxically as they knew, was also overflowing fullness.

Philosophy professor Troy Wilson Organ writes that for the Indians and yogis, zero is essentially a "productive point of potentiality," a "fertile seed" ready to take root and blossom.[2] German Indologist Betty Heimann, one of the early pioneers in comparative philosophy, seconds this: "Zero is the productive All and None, the matrix of positive and negative, of addition and subtraction, of generating and destroying capacities. It is the productive point of indifference and balance. It is the no-more- and not-yet-distinct thing."[3]

We might say then that zero is both the focus and expression of the yogis' tireless quest for the Self, which they call Atman-Brahman. Renu Jain, a professor of mathematics at Jiwaji University in Gwalior, affirms that the idea of "spiritual nothingness" led to mathematical zero, adding that the "word used in philosophical texts to mean nothing, or the void, is 'shunya,' the same word later used to mean zero."[4]

▸ ▸ STORY

How Shunya *Became* Zero

Words, like living things, change and mature over time, and we can frequently learn something important, even surprising, about the "adult" word by investigating its birth and youth. When I traced our word *zero* back to its source through its French, Italian, and Latin ancestors, I came at last to an Arabic word, *sifr*, which means "nothing, cipher" (cipher being another English word for *zero*).

It was rather curious, after seeing three expected European-language ancestors, to come face-to-face with what was an unexpected Arabic word. I suspected there was something behind this story, and so there was. Around 770 CE, a visiting Indian scholar told the caliph of Baghdad about the groundbreaking work of our Brahmagupta. The scholar had with him a copy of Brahmagupta's book, written in Sanskrit about 140 years earlier, and the caliph commissioned a translation. When the translator came to the Sanskrit word *shunya*, one of the two words Brahmagupta used for zero (the other being *kha*), he rendered it into Arabic as *sifr*. So every time we say "zero," we can hear a faint echo of *shunya*.

◂ ◂

BRAHMAN: ALL AND NONE

Before they reach it [i.e., Brahman], words turn back
Together with the mind . . .
Taittiriya Upanishad 2.9.1

Who or what is Brahman? We begin with a story.

▸ ▸ STORY

Bahva Teaches Vashkali about Brahman

One day Vashkali approached his teacher, Bahva, and asked, "Please teach me, most reverent sir, the nature of Brahman." He then waited humbly for the response. Silence. After a few minutes, Vashkali thought maybe Bahva hadn't heard his question. So again he respectfully asked, "Please, sir, teach me the nature of Brahman," and again with bowed head waited for the teacher's response. But as before, a long silence. Undeterred, the student asked a third time, and for the third time the only answer was silence. Feeling a bit hurt by his teacher's continued silence, Vashkali asked, "Please, sir, why won't you teach me about the nature of Brahman?" Bahva looked at Vashkali and smiled. "I have been teaching you," he said softly, "but you don't understand."

◂ ◂

In asking "Who or what is Brahman?" it occurred to me that I should perhaps follow Bahva's lead and remain silent myself, leaving the rest of this page blank and moving on to chapter 2. After all, if Bahva—undoubtedly a realized yogi—had nothing to say about Brahman, how can I, in my Self-ignorance, even dare to try? What can anyone say about Brahman, from which all words and the mind "turn back" before they get anywhere close? To whittle that down to what it means in one word, Brahman is *ineffable*, which the dictionary defines as "incapable of being expressed."

But I have to say something about Brahman because after all, as Professor Heinrich Zimmer has noted, it "has been from Vedic times to the present day the most important single concept of Hindu religion and philosophy,"[5] though I'm not sure we can use the word *concept* about an "it" that's far beyond all conceptualization.

So despite my misgivings, I'll take on the question of what Brahman is. It's one that receives a good deal of attention in Indian spiritual literature, particularly that produced in the school of Vedanta, which we'll go into in chapter 2. There's no agreement on how *Brahman* should be rendered into English, if at all. It's one of those Sanskrit words, like *dharma* and *karma*, that translators tend to leave alone. Probably the most common English rendering is "the Absolute" (always with a capital *A*). Though this is more of an interpretation than a translation, its definition as "perfect, unqualified, unlimited, pure" provides a clear snapshot of Brahman's nature.

A few scholars have made valiant attempts to find an English equivalent for Brahman based on its root, *brih*, "to grow, expand." Georg Feuerstein proposes the "vast expanse"; Alain Danielou, "the Immensity." Whatever we decide to call Brahman, it's important to remember that the word itself is a neuter noun, and so the proper pronoun is "it," never "he" or "she." We should also be careful not to confuse Brahman with its final *n*, with Brahma, the creator deity of the Hindu *trimurti*, or "triple form" or trinity, which is a masculine noun and so a "he."

There are two more things that may be of interest with the name Brahman. If we go to the entry for *shunya* in the Apte Sanskrit-English dictionary, we find one definition as "the name of Brahman." Here we have a curious paradox involving the roots of both *shunya*, which is *shvi*, and *Brahman* with *brih*. They mean almost the same thing: "to increase." So here we have *shunya*, "zero, void," rooted in a verb that means "to increase," and *Brahman*, which has been interpreted as "immensity," with an alternate name which means "void." This certainly seems to be an example of what Professor Heimann had to say about the paradoxical nature of zero in Indian culture, that it's the "matrix" of both "the All" and "the None."

▸ ▸ BEHIND THE NUMBERS

Purna

Another example of the Indian's embrace of "the All and the None" is the word *purna*. It generally means "full, all, entire," but the very last words in its dictionary definition read, "the cipher or figure 0." Like *zero*, *cipher* is also rooted in the Arabic *sifr*, and so *shunya*.

◂ ◂

Finally, the name itself presents us with a problem. As we read in the quote at the head of this section, words and the mind "turn back" from ineffable Brahman. No word can describe it, and since *brahman* is a word, then Brahman actually has no name; in fact, one of its nicknames is "nameless" (*anamaka*), though of course "nameless" is also a name and a word.

To complete our portrait of Brahman, we'll turn to the 20 or 21 texts known as the Yoga Upanishads, generally written in the fourteenth and fifteenth centuries CE. If we run a search for *brahman* through the collection's 500 pages, we get a response of nearly 500 citations.

What we find confirms what we've already gathered from the etymological excavation of *absolute*. Brahman is free of any and all conditions or limitations, including space and time, it's "beginningless and . . . endless."[6] It's ultimately the source or "Prime cause,"[7] the "Supreme Consciousness" that manifests itself as the universe. "All is absolutely the Brahman alone."[8]

TWO "FORMS" OF BRAHMAN: WITHOUT QUALITIES (*NIRGUNA*) AND WITH (*SAGUNA*)

There are two forms of brahman, the shaped and the unshaped, the mortal and the immortal, the still and the moving, the present and the beyond.

Brihadaranyanka Upanishad 2.3.1

I should immediately note that the heading of this subsection is quite misleading, which is a common problem whenever trying to say anything about Brahman. As the Upanishad forewarns us, trying to reach "it" in word or thought is futile; our words and thoughts will "turn back" and fall to Earth. As a consequence, we have to imagine there are two Brahmans. One is *nirguna* Brahman, "without (*nir*) qualities or attributes (*guna*)," and so is qualified with a string of words each suffixed with *-less*: formless, changeless, partless, beginningless, and endless. This Brahman is, in a word, transcendent; it exists "beyond" the universe—as impossible as that is for us to conceive. To us, nirguna appears indistinguishable from nothing, from zero. But like zero, nirguna isn't nothing; rather, it's nothing we can know because it's the source of knowing, the ultimate subject, the "knower" of everything which itself can't be known.

I suppose I need to backtrack a bit from the contention that nothing can be said about nirguna. In fact, it's often characterized by the phrase *saccidananda*, which is a combination of three words, *sat*, *cit*, and *ananda*. Simply, *sat* means "being, existing," but we can also add to this that it's "real, true, good, beautiful, wise, honest." Brahman then, as sat (pronounced sut), is the ultimate ground of being, the foundation underlying the universe. *Cit* literally means "to perceive, observe." It's the light of consciousness without which our world would be blacked out. Finally there's *ananda* (pronounced AH-nan-duh), usually rendered as "bliss." (Remember always to put the emphasis here on the first syllable; uh-NAN-duh, the way it's usually pronounced, means just the opposite, "joyless.") Ananda has nothing to do with the feelings we typically get from pleasurable experiences. We come to share in this bliss "to the extent that we are or become self-complete; our pleasures are fleeting expressions of the joy that is our very nature."[9]

While nirguna transcends our world, *saguna* Brahman, "with (*sa*) qualities or attributes (*guna*)," is everywhere at our fingertips; that is, it's immanent in our world. Nirguna is the totally passive witness (*sakshin*) of the tragicomedy we call the universe; saguna is "that from which the origin, subsistence, and dissolution of this world proceed."[10] These are the same three actions we'll find parceled out among the three members of the Hindu *trimurti* or "triple form" of deities (Brahma, Vishnu, and Shiva), or for the Shaivites, Shiva alone. We might tend to look more favorably on saguna than nirguna, since the former is our creator and sustainer, though admittedly, it's the power that also reabsorbs the world at the end of its current cycle.

There's a question that's frequently asked about Brahman: if it's transcendent and complete in itself and so needs nothing, why does it need to create a universe? The answer is that it doesn't create out of desire, as most of us do when we create something, but from an excess of joy in a spirit of "play" (*lila*). "Although the creation of this world appears to us a weighty and difficult undertaking," writes the sage Shankara, "it is mere play to the Lord, whose power is unlimited."[11]

ATMAN-BRAHMAN: "ESSENCE"

The essence of the entire visible universe is denoted by the word Brahman. That Brahman is of the nature of the self-luminous Atman.

Pancadashi 5.8

As we'll soon see, the universe has two forms, the macrocosm (or "Brahma egg") and the microcosm (or "ball egg"). The former is the universe at large; the latter is its tiny replica, which is each one of us (see p. 33). Similarly, Brahman has macro and micro versions: the former is called Brahman; the latter, Atman, which is the "essence" of Brahman in each of us. Once again, as we often find in yoga, embedded as we are in dualist consciousness (see p. 24), we need two words to talk about what's ultimately one existent —at least according to Vedanta (again see p. 16)—which we can call Atman-Brahman (like the Absolute for Brahman with its capital *A*, the Self for Atman is spelled with a capital *S*).

Technically Atman, the Self, also has two forms, analogous to those of Brahman: the transcendent or the "supreme Self" (*paramatman*), indistinguishable from Brahman, and the immanent or embodied or "living" Self, the *jiva* or *jivatman*.

Unlike the neuter noun *Brahman*, *Atman* is masculine, though this gender seems to raise a contradiction. If Atman is equivalent to Brahman, properly then, Atman should be referred to as "it." We find that in the singular, *Atman* can be used as a reflexive pronoun for "all three persons and all three genders," according to the Sanskrit-English dictionary. So we'll keep things neutral and also refer to Atman as "it."

Atman's root is uncertain. The favored possibility is *an*, "to breathe" (also the root of *prana*), though the dictionary also proposes *at*, "to roam or wander," and *va*, "to blow." Eventually the word "came to be applied to whatever constitutes the essential part of anything," particularly the Self.[12] Don't be misled by the two names. Though each of these words began with its own independent significance—Brahman as the source and sustainer of the universe, Atman as the inner Self—they eventually became synonymous and made the equation Brahman equals Atman.

▸ ▸ PRACTICE

"Not This, Not This" (Neti Neti)

As we'll see in chapter 10, there are maybe two dozen sayings (*vakya*) that have been drawn from the Upanishads (see p. 17) for use as platforms for meditation. Some are very short—no more than three words—and others are full sentences. Four in particular have been singled out as "great sayings" (*maha vakya*). Probably the shortest and simplest of the sayings not included among the great four is "not this, not this" (*neti neti*).

"Not this, not this" means there's no positive language that can in any way adequately describe Brahman, because it transcends all name and form. But although it's impossible to say what Brahman is, we can say a good deal about what it's not—and that's the thrust of neti neti: Brahman isn't this and it isn't that. As with all of these vakya, neti neti is a focus for meditation, but its use needn't be limited to a formal sitting practice. We can apply it to whatever we encounter during a normal day, a constant reminder that Brahman isn't limited to any one thing or things, no matter how immense or minute. This doesn't imply that our world is an illusion, quite the contrary. Brahman is the "single Subject of the universe," and it inhabits "*all* things."[13]

Of course, alternately, you may be more disposed to affirming the presence of Brahman everywhere you look. In this case, break *neti* down into its two constituents, *na iti*, drop the negative *na*, and then whatever you see is *iti iti*, "this, this."

◂ ◂

To me, no matter how unthinkable all this about Brahman seems to us, the most important thing to remember is that, regardless of who we are, Brahman is always with us. It's the "silent witness," the "witness of all";[14]

whatever we experience in our lives and however we react to those experiences, we're grounded in the Absolute. We sometimes imagine that so-called higher consciousness is beyond our reach, that it's only accessible to dedicated yogis, but that's mistaken. Higher consciousness is simply consciousness: it's who we are, 24/7, awake, asleep, and at all points in between. All that is required to realize it is to take a figurative step back from everything, including your self (with a small *s*), and observe without judgment or expectation. That's Brahman. Easy? Maybe not long term at first, but surely it can be done over time with persistence and one baby step at a time.

2

INDIAN PHILOSOPHY BY THE NUMBERS

Monism, Dualism, Triadism or Trika

The manifold universe is, in truth, a single Reality. There is only that one Great Being, which the sages call *brahman*, in which all the countless forms of existence reside. That Great Being is utter Consciousness, and it is the very essence, of Self (*atman*), of all beings.

Georg Feuerstein, "That Art Thou,"
The Deeper Dimensions of Yoga

Monism, dualism, and triadism are the basic one, two, three of Indian philosophy. The question they propose to answer concerns the nature of our reality and our relationship to it: does that reality emerge from a single source (monism), result from the interplay of two distinct existents (dualism), or arise, somehow, in some unique and creative way, as a combination of both (triadism)? And what about us? How do we fit into each of these realities, and what determines a successful outcome for our participation?

MONISM

The word *monism* comes from the Greek *monos*, "single." We can sum this doctrine up quite neatly as "All is One." For Hindu monists, this means everything that makes up the universe, whether living or not, can be resolved back into a single source, usually called Brahman (or *paramatman*), which ultimately is no different than our own Self, usually called Atman (or *jivatman*). "Just as no differences exist when water is thrown into water, milk into milk . . . , similarly there remains no difference between the Jivatman and the Paramatman."[1]

Monism may make a kind of sense in theory, but when we try to put some flesh on its bones in our day-to-day experience, it makes no sense at all. Though it assures us that the manifold universe is a single reality, including each of us in some way in the mix, that's certainly not how most of us encounter that reality. If I look out my window at the street I live on, I see houses, trees, power poles, parked cars, people walking their dogs, kids riding their bikes or roller-skating—in sum, none of this appears in the least to be one "great being," nor do I feel that I myself share in its essence, whatever that is.

The best I can do is narrow it all down to me and not-me—that is, everything and everyone else. In truth, it's dualism that makes sense to us: we feel right at home with twoness, but oneness leaves us scratching our heads. For the monist this proves one thing about us: we and our view of the world are under the sway of humanity's age-old bugaboo Self-ignorance (*avidya*)—the mistaken belief that we are who we're not and not who we are, a severe limitation in our capacity not only for Self-knowledge, but for knowing the world as it truly is as well. We'll return to avidya in later chapters.

The best-known monistic Indian philosophy is Vedanta, of which there are several subschools. There is, I think, a touch of irony in this: that even a doctrine promoting the oneness of all is fractured into competing stances regarding what that oneness is like. *Vedanta* literally means the "end (*anta*) of the veda," this latter word rooted in *vid*, "to know," from which we get English words like *video* and *vision*, as well as Sanskrit *avidya*, "to not know." This phrase has a backstory.

▸ ▸ BEHIND THE NUMBERS

Vedanta: The End of the Veda

The Veda—literally, "knowledge"—is a sprawling collection of texts that hold a special place in Indian spiritual literature. The knowledge preserved in these texts is revered as *shruti* ("that which is heard"), sacred knowledge received from Brahman by a coterie of seers, usually seven in number, at the beginning of each world cycle. Four texts compose the foundation of the Veda, the oldest and most important being the *Rig Veda* (RV), the "knowledge of praise" (*ric*), which consists of just over a thousand mantra-poems. It's quite difficult, if not impossible, to date the RV's age with any certainty. Most scholars estimate it to be around 3,500 years, but this is contested. Feuerstein dates it back 5,000 years. No matter, say the Indian pandits, since the Veda is delivered to humankind at the start of each world cycle, it hasn't any age—it's eternal.

My copy of the RV (and like most of these texts, it's available online in English translation), which includes an extensive commentary, runs to about 650 pages of what appears to be 8- or 9-point type. I mention this because the RV existed before the Indians had invented writing. In order to preserve its wisdom through time, Hindu priests memorized the entire text word for word and passed it on orally with hardly any variation from generation to generation for hundreds of years. I always think of this remarkable feat when I put down my house keys somewhere and then can't find them five minutes later.

The "end of the Veda" actually refers to the group of texts called the Upanishads, generally dated between 800 and 300 BCE, appended to the tail end of one of the four foundation texts. Most scholars interpret "the end" in two senses: first, as the physical tail end of the collection; and second, in the sense of the final goal of the teaching. A few scholars, though, see the early Upanishads as representing a completely new direction of the Vedic teaching, so for them, these texts mark the end of the earlier teaching.

▸ ▸ BEHIND THE NUMBERS

"You Say You Want a Revolution?": *The Internalization of the Vedic Ritual*

The "new direction" in Vedic teaching represented (according to some scholars) by the Upanishads marks the first great revolution in the history of yoga, which involved the internalization or sublimation of the external Vedic ritual. As I understand it—and to describe it as simply as possible—there came a time when the outward ritual of fire altars and sacrifices to the gods, which expected a suitable return on the sacrificial "investment," lost its original meaning and power, and a kind of spiritual hunger then set in among certain members of the priestly and ruling classes, who transferred the "external performance" of the Vedic ritual to an "internal meditation." As Paul Deussen suggests, the "true sacrifice becomes the fire oblation on the breath (*pranagnihotra*)." The Self is now both the sacrificer and the sacrificial offering; the many "sacrificial utensils," parts of the body—"the right hand the Sruva ladle," "the left hand the pot of clarified butter." Now the "real purpose of the rite is not its external performance" and gaining the gods' favor, but "knowledge of its deeper meaning . . . , which points to an underlying foundation or being" on which the entire universal edifice, including of course ourselves, rests.[2] The Vedantins call this foundation or being "Brahman."

◂ ◂

Vedanta is based on a trio of texts collectively known as "three ways to attain" (*prasthana traya*). Along with the Upanishads, there's the *Vedanta Sutra* VS (or *Brahma Sutra*) by Badarayana of the second century BCE and the world-famous *Bhagavad Gita* (BG) of the third or fourth century BCE.

The oldest surviving subschool of Vedanta is known as *Advaita*, a word that consists of the prefix *a-*, "not," and *dvaita*, "duality," and so means "nonduality, having no duplicate; sole, unique." According to historian of religion Mircea Eliade, Vedanta is organized around four "kinetic ideas":[3]

1. The law of universal causality or action (*karma*), which binds us to the unending round of birth-death-rebirth, known as *samsara*— literally "wandering through." We might imagine that repeated lives might be an interesting, if not always entirely pleasant way to spend eternity, but for the early yogis the universe was a burdensome vale of tears, the release from which was the primary goal of their efforts. The seventeenth-century *Gheranda Samhita* (GS) compared *samsara* to a waterwheel: just as the wheel with its buckets "revolves up and down, driven by cows," so our Self "wanders through births and deaths," driven by karma.[4]

2. Cosmic illusion or *maya*, the mysterious process that gives birth to and maintains the entire universe. *Maya* is sometimes identified with *avidya*, which has two powers: concealment (*avarana*) of the unity of Atman and Brahman, which sets up a false duality, and the projection (*vikshepa*) of the endless diversity of the universe, which lures us into identifying our unlimited Self with material limitations (*upadhis*). The consequence is *duhkha*, literally "uneasiness, pain, sorrow."

3. An absolute reality, called Brahman, that transcends cosmic illusion and all human experience, and yet is no different than the individual Self (*Atman*).

4. The means to realize the Self and gain liberation (*moksha*), otherwise known as yoga. The first surviving concrete mention of yoga practice occurs in the *Katha Upanishad* (KU) of the fourth or fifth century BCE:

When the senses are firmly reined in,
that is Yoga, so people think.
From distractions a man is then free,
for Yoga is the coming-into-being,
as well as the ceasing-to-be.[5]

Liberation here is not a union in the usual sense of the word, in which "two or more things," typically the Self and Brahman, are joined together. This isn't possible in a monist environment, because the supposed split between these two existents is due to misapprehension. Brahman and Atman are for all intents and purposes the same, and have been and will be through all time. Yoga instead *reveals* this eternal union, which means too that yoga isn't a "path," as it is so frequently described, because there's nowhere to go: we already are where we want to be, but we just don't know it.

A question is often asked about maya and cosmic illusion: is the world real or is it a very real-seeming illusion? The answer depends on our perspective. Advaita posits two levels of truth: the relative and the absolute. With the former, if I stub my barefoot toe on a rock, then yes, the world unquestioningly exists as I hop around on one foot, cursing. But when the truth is absolute, then the world is a superimposition, an *adhyaropa*, a "wrong attribution" of something unreal to the Real—that is, Brahman. If we could see it through the eyes of an "insightful Vedanta master," remarks an early Advaitin Gauda Pada, our world would be nothing but "dreams, illusions and fairy cities in the skies."[6]

Are we unreal too then? Not exactly, though I wouldn't get overly attached to the person on your driver's license, with its disastrous mug shot, the purple-streaked hair, and lowballed weight, because that person is also a relative truth. If we could see the absolute truth about ourselves, we'd understand that the person we think we are is something like a superimposition, an "imposition" on our Self. We would also understand this Self is nothing else than utter consciousness, the distilled essence of Brahman.

As I mentioned, the Advaitins have split over doctrinal issues into squabbling subschools. They do see eye to eye on the basics, however: the single reality of Atman-Brahman and the ultimate unreality of everything else, the world as an illusion projected onto Brahman like a movie on a movie screen, and the force of Self-ignorance that binds us to the illusion.

At the same time, the Advaitins disagree about that ignorance. The question is posed: if ignorance is the cause of both our bondage and the illusion concealing the truth about the world, who exactly is it that's ignorant? One school suggests that it's Brahman itself. But then another school responds, quite logically, that if Brahman's essence is knowledge, it's contradictory to maintain it can be affected by ignorance.

So ignorance is something other than but not separate from Brahman. It can't be, for if there's something in the world that isn't Brahman, then Advaita would collapse. Here's the paradox: We know ignorance exists, but at the same time it's not Brahman that's ignorant. But everything that exists must exist under Brahman's aegis. The Vedantins then come to the only conclusion left to them: Self-ignorance is inexplicable.

▸ ▸ BEHIND THE NUMBERS

One in Sanskrit

The Sanskrit word for one is *eka*. In the yoga lexicon, words prefixed with *eka* are legion. Its widespread presence reflects the great importance Hindu culture and yoga place on the underlying oneness of ourselves and the universe. Eka stands for "unity, singleness, one without a second." This is also, of course, the very definition of yoga. Eka further expresses exclusiveness, preeminence, either by nature or by choice (*ekata, ekatva*). It's *that* one only and it happens only once; so it's unique, excellent, without peer, matchless, chief among the numbers, sincere and truthful.

The One is our refuge (*ekashraya*), our delight (*ekarata*). We can rest in it with devotion (*ekabhakta, ekapara*) or in our thoughts (*ekamati*), and there know the essence of truth (*ekarasa*). When we see the "diversity of all beings" as "resting in the One" (*ekastha*), and from "That alone spreading out," then we'll attain Brahman.[7] This is ultimately the "one aim" (*ekanta*) we have on Earth.

In practice, eka excludes everything but the one thing held in consciousness (*ekamanas, ekasarga*). It's one-pointed, closely attentive, absorbed in (*ekagra, ekabhuta, ekacita*); it gazes fixedly at (*ekadrishti*). As a name for the seed mantra OM, it's the one imperishable, unalterable syllable (*ekakshara*) that wise ones call the "supreme effulgence."[8]

The yogi wanders (*ekacara*) and lives alone (*ekaka*) in a "secluded hut" (*ekanta matha*). An ascetic follower of Vishnu (a Vaishnava) generally carries a single staff and so is known as an *eka dandin*. The staff tells the world that he has "control over the ever unsteady and fickle consciousness (*citta*)," which though one, "assumes various forms."[9] In regard to asana, the yogis have purportedly whittled down the original 8.4 million taught by Shiva ultimately to a much more manageable one.

Deities also have nicknames that begin with *eka*. Ganesha, the popular elephant-headed god, is revered as a remover of obstacles. He lost one of his tusks in a tussle with another god, or in another tale, broke off a tusk to use as a pen to write the *Mahabharata* (MaB), as it was dictated by Vyasa. Because of this, however it happened, he's known as "One Tooth" (*eka danta*) or "One Tusk" (*eka rada*).

The *Vishnu Sahasranama* lists, as the title indicates, 1,000 names (*sahasra nama*) for Vishnu. Eka, "The One," is his 725th name; "One Self" (*ekatman*) is his 965th name. He's also known as "One Horn" (*ekashringa*), the horn (*shringa*) signifying the "height or perfection of anything," "self-reliance or strength," and a "being of singular eminence."

Shiva is said to have 1,008 nicknames. He's the "One Light" (*eka jyoti*) and the "One Garmented Lord" (*ekambara ishvara*). There's a play on words here. *Ambara* means both "garment" and "sky," which implies that Shiva is "wearing the sky"; that is to say, as is common among Indian ascetics, he's naked. There are several names that refer to his famous third eye.

In the end there's one God (*ekadeva*), but still and all, eka is surprisingly "little" and "small."

◀ ◀

THE FOURFOLD MEANS (*SADHANA*)

Four, the number of the earth, represents the fulfillment of manifestations in all the spheres of existence, the four stages that may be found in every form of development, of life.

Alain Danielou, *The Gods of India*

The fourfold means of traditional Advaita Vedanta practice are collectively known as Jnana Yoga. *Jnana* is often defined as "higher" wisdom, but "higher" can be misleading. It suggests we have to climb some kind of a spiritual ladder to reach the wisdom that is somehow "above" or "beyond" us. At the same time, it also suggests worldly wisdom is "lower"—that thousands of years of hard-earned learning in areas like physics and mathematics, medicine, psychology, and the arts are somehow less meaningful and essential to our lives.

Moreover, because "higher wisdom" is believed to be "out of reach," it's often portrayed as something rare and inaccessible to the average person. But in fact, that wisdom is *who we are*, our Self, our very being, and so-called lower wisdom is an expression of that Self. No doubt its realization requires a strong and sustained effort to achieve, as does much of worldly wisdom, but it's an effort well within most everyone's capability. It's always right in the figurative palm of our hand.

Vedanta recommends these means to attain moksha, lasting liberation:

1. The nonstop discrimination (*viveka*) between what's eternal and what's transient;
2. Renunciation (*vairagya*) of the transient and any benefits derived from the fruits of our actions;
3. Practice of the six fulfillments (*shat sampatti*): tranquility (*shama*), self-restraint (*dama*), withdrawal from worldly interests (*uparati*), endurance or forbearance (*titiksha*), faith (*shraddha*), freedom from conflicts (*samadhana*);
4. And most importantly, the unquenchable urge toward liberation (*mumukshutva*).

Though we may all have the capability, what we don't all have is the burning "desire for liberation" (*mumukshu*). Make no mistake, just as wisdom is innate in each of us, so is the desire to be Self-realized, though it affects different people in different ways. We might compare *mumukshu* to what Patanjali calls "excitement, intensity, vehemence" (*samvega*, from *vega*, "impetus, outburst of passion, current of tears"), of which there are three levels of intensity that describe three types of student: mild (*mridu*), medium (*madhya*), and above measure, excessive (*adhimatra*).[10] Apparently, as the intensity of the yogi's practice efforts rise, the sooner those efforts will yield the desired result.

These three additional practices are also associated with Jnana Yoga:

1. Listening (*shravana*) to the study/discussion of the Upanishads and the teaching of the guru (stresses tradition)
2. Pondering (*manana*) over what is heard (stresses intellect)
3. Meditation (*nididhyasana*) on the realization "I am Brahman" (*aham brahma asmi*) (stresses insight)

Even with the capability and red-hot desire for liberation, there was no guarantee that a traditional aspirant's hopes would be realized. That's because there was one crucial element without which each and every aspirant was doomed to fail, and that's the guru. "The Guru alone is the ultimate limit; the Guru alone is the highest wealth. For the reason that he teaches That, therefore is the Guru greater than all else."[11]

It was unquestioningly believed that a guru was an indispensable access point to Atman-Brahman. He not only provided guidance and support to the aspirant, but more importantly, he was an unlimited source of transformative power that could, with a look, a touch, or a word, connect the aspirant straight to the Self. We'll return to the guru in chapter 6.

DUALISM (*DVAITA*)

[Classical (Patanjali) Yoga] seems to be . . . concerned with the way the world and its phenomena are essentially seen by the ordinary individual. Our everyday experiences do not point to a unity of any kind. I experience everything essentially as a contrast, a separateness, between myself and other people.

Nandini Iyer, "'It Ain't Necessarily So,'"
in Knut Jacobsen, ed., *Theory and Practice of Yoga:*
Essays in Honour of Gerald James Larson

When you wake up in the morning and look around your room, what's the first thing you notice about what you see in relation to yourself, even though it's likely not be a conscious thought? It might be that everything within the compass of your vision is not you, no matter how far out you expand your vision. Even if you could see to the edge of the known universe, whatever you see will always be other than you. The separation is physical, of course, "you" are "in here," in your body, encased in 206 bones wrapped in a two-millimeter-thick sheath of skin, and everyone and everything else is "out there," outside of your body.

But there's something else that sets you apart. To a greater or lesser degree, you can know yourself—your likes and dislikes, your habits, your personal history—but you can never know the other like you know yourself. Just as you will always be you, the other will always be other. Looked at in this way, we're both utterly unique and utterly alone in the universe. We might call this two-ism, or if we're of a more philosophic mindset, a simple form of dualism, that we experience everything essentially as a separateness between me and not-me.

Patanjali's version of dualism digs a bit deeper into our very being. As he tells it, our true Self, purusha, is analogous to "me" when we wake in the morning, the observer. Now though, in addition to all the furniture in the room, our body, which is made of the same stuff as our nightstand or chest of drawers, is also on the "outside," another "not-me," however much we value our mortal coil. But he doesn't stop there.

Philosophers and other big thinkers have been trying to explain human consciousness for many hundreds of years, but no one has yet come up with a story that satisfies everyone. I personally believe that consciousness can't be explained for the very simple reason that it doesn't want to—that at least some aspect of it wants to remain a mystery to encourage us humans to keep asking questions and searching for answers. But that's just me. Patanjali has it that our consciousness is the product of the two eternals in his universe: purusha or immaterial sentience and prakriti or insentient matter. You might be somewhat surprised by the idea that consciousness, at least in part, is a material process. When I look across my room at my beloved guitar, my consciousness literally takes on the shape of that instrument. But I wouldn't know it unless the "light" of purusha shined through that shape so that I recognized it as "guitar."

At the same time, if that material process didn't exist, there would be nothing to shape itself as the things and people around me, and purusha could know nothing of the world since it has no agency of its own. Human consciousness then has a material foundation, extremely subtle matter to be sure, but matter all the same, illuminated by the Self, which Patanjali significantly calls the *drashtir*, the "seer." It reminds us of the comment of the English mystic-poet William Blake that (and I paraphrase), I don't see with my eyes, I see through them. For Patanjali then, purusha is the true seer, and our eyes are the means by which it sees—and our limbs are the means by which it moves through and handles the world, our nose how it smells, ears how it hears, and so on. Patanjali's brand of dualism finishes the retreat inward. Not only is the body on the "outside" when we wake up in the morning, so too now is the material "ground" of our consciousness.

▸ ▸ PRACTICE

The Seer (Drashtir) *and a Kaleidoscope*

One way I've found to help me visualize how the seer illuminates nature is by looking through a kaleidoscope. I imagine most everyone has, at one time or another, peered through the peephole at one end of these tube-shaped toys. When we turn the tube, little pieces of colored glass or plastic contained in its far end tumble around and around, and are transformed by inclined mirrors into countless shapes and patterns. We are of course irresistibly drawn to the "beautiful forms," and as a result we forget one important thing: without the light shining through the far end of the tube, we'd see nothing.

When I look at the people and things in the world, I imagine them to be the little colored pieces of glass, tumbling around as the world turns. Naturally my first inclination is to identify with all the interesting and alluring shapes and patterns created by the world-kaleidoscope. But I can shift my perspective and identify with the light of the seer shining through me, illuminating whatever I'm observing. Then I can swing back and forth between the two positions: me in the world, frolicking with all the beautiful shapes and patterns, and then me, now the seer, watching the world go tumbling by.

◂ ◂

Now there's one very sticky sticking point regarding the contact between matter and Self. We've undeniable proof that our two existents interact: if they didn't, the world wouldn't, couldn't, exist.

But Patanjali insists that his dualism is absolute, that there's no real connection between Self and matter. This strict dualism, as Georg Feuerstein writes, gives rise to a "serious philosophical problem. For, if there is no real link between the Being-Awareness which is the Self and the unconscious conglomeration of elements which is the organism—how can the Self be said to induce consciousness?"[12]

Patanjali's solution isn't entirely convincing to committed skeptics such as myself. It seems that his "strict dualism" isn't quite strictly strict. Apparently the light of the Self is "reflected" in the most refined aspect of our citta, known as the *buddhi*, usually translated as "intellect" with its high content of the sattva "strand" (*guna*; for more on this see p. 36).

Professor of Hindu philosophy and religion Edwin Bryant, who for me is the most levelheaded and accessible commentator on Patanjali, explains that Patanjali, who inherited this dualism from earlier teachings known as Samkhya ("enumeration"), isn't writing a philosophical treatise, so the metaphysics of all "manifest reality," including the question of how the two existents interact, is unimportant.[13] Patanjali's initial concern is presenting a relationship between the yogi and the world that's easily understood and accepted, so the yogi gets the practice off on the right foot.

This brings us back to our basic dualism, except that the identities of me and not-me are redefined as *purusha* and *prakriti* respectively.

Feuerstein sums this up succinctly: "Philosophically unattractive," he admits, but "of considerable practical relevance."[14]

If we ask a fairly well-informed student for an English translation of the Sanskrit term *yoga*, we'll likely get as a response the reasonably accurate "union." This word is derived from the root *yuj*, meaning "to yoke, join." But as Gerald Larson explains, there are two yuj roots, and the second simply means "disciplined meditation."[15] This is the source and meaning of the word *yoga* as it's used in the YS. We'll talk more about this later, but for now remember, at the culmination of Patanjali's practice, no matter what you've read in some modern interpretations of the YS, *there's no union.* As we'll see, it's quite the opposite: there's a final *dis*-union, and Patanjali Yoga is more properly called *vi-yoga*, literally "away from (vi) union (yoga)." As Feuerstein notes, "For Patanjali . . . liberation means total isolation from the world. . . . In other words, the practitioner's absolute withdrawal from the phenomenal reality, in its visible and invisible dimensions."[16]

▸ ▸ BEHIND THE NUMBERS

Two in Sanskrit

The Sanskrit word for two is *dvi* (in compounds prefixing other words, *dvi* becomes *dva*). Where *eka* is one-without-a-second and so conflict-free, *dvi* is a continual confrontation between polar opposites. In the yoga of Patanjali, there's a kind of cooperative opposition between the system's principal elements, matter (*prakriti*) and Self (*purusha*), a worldview known as dualism (*dvaita*). Patanjali literally calls them "two-twos" (*dvandva*), which can be rendered as "pairs of opposites." A dvandva can be any "two-two": a pair, a couple, male and female, even the twins of the zodiac sign Gemini. In the Hatha tradition, the pair may be having a "fight, quarrel," and because of this they may need protection from each other, and so *dvandva* also means "stronghold, fortress." Such pairs of opposites are scattered throughout the Hatha Yoga tradition as teaching tools. One example is the story of the bird and the ant from the *Varaha Upanishad* (VU).

◂ ◂

▸ ▸ STORY

The Bird and the Ant

> He who adopts the course pursued by the bird (Shuka) attains liberation, as also he who adopts the course of the ant (Vamadeva).
>
> *Varaha Upanishad* 4.2.34

The ultimate purpose of just about every traditional yoga school is the reorientation of our identity away from the inherent Self-limitations and resultant existential suffering of our ego-dominated consciousness to our eternal, blissful "authentic" self. The way to accomplish this varies to a greater or lesser degree from school to school, but according to the VU, all of those ways will ultimately follow one of two paths laid out by the gods. Today we might call them the fast and slow tracks, but the anonymous author of this text calls them each by two names: one an ancient sage, the other a living creature.

The "fast" path of the two is that of Shuka (literally "parrot"), or the Bird. This is, if I understand it correctly, the path of the ascetic, who makes a purposeful effort to gain liberation in the current life. Several techniques are mentioned as conducive to that goal, among them the practice of *samadhi* (as taught in Patanjali Yoga), the study of the truth embodied in the great sayings (*maha vakya*, see chapter 9) drawn from the books of the Veda, and through the "method of exclusion"—that is, the continual application of the formula (or mantra) "not this, not this" (*neti neti*; see chapter 2). This latter will ideally lead to our "freedom from the known," as Jiddu Krishnamurti once put it, the complete detachment of our identity from everything in this world not Brahman (see chapter 2).

The "slow" path is named after Vamadeva ("left-hand deity"), or the Ant. This seems to be the practice of the everyday person—that is, most of us. Without question we're strongly committed to our practice, but not as fully and irrevocably as were the ascetic yogis when this text was written hundreds of years ago. Imagine giving up everything, your entire world, to embark on a search through unknown territory where danger lurked around every corner and with no guarantee that you'd ever achieve your goal.

We've all seen a lonely ant making its way across a desk or kitchen table. The desk I'm sitting at now is two feet wide: to an ant—if my calculations are correct—that's the equivalent of an American football field from the *end* of one end zone to the end of the other, over 120 yards. On the slow path, we're like the ant standing at one edge of my desk and gazing out across a vast white field strewn with obstacles: pencils, books, my keyboard, all appearing to the ant many times larger than they appear to us. And there's always the ultimate danger, of which the ant is blissfully unaware, of some impersonal godlike power unthinkingly crushing it under its thumb.

Yet the anonymous Varaha author assures us ants we'll attain liberation.

◂ ◂

TRIADISM (*TRIKA*)

As we've seen, monism posits that the entire universe with all its dizzying diversity can finally be resolved back into one unifying existent, usually called Atman-Brahman. Dualism, on the other hand, rejects that position and counters that the universe is instead the outcome of the interaction, however that's possible, between two entirely distinct existents, one of them completely material (*prakriti*), the other completely immaterial (*purusha*). The monist's salvation involves some form of the Self's reintegration with the Absolute; the dualist's, a complete abandonment of any association with matter.

It's safe to say that neither of these systems is perfect. The monist has difficulty explaining how the power of maya fits into its all-is-one universe; the dualist has a hard time justifying the interaction between its two supposedly radically separate existents. Would a kind of meeting of the minds be possible between these two systems, combining the best of both? The answer is a resounding yes.

The third system is called various things. Since its origin is traced to Kashmir in northwestern India 1,200 to 1,300 years ago—though scholars agree its rudiments can be pushed back a few more centuries—and since it's dedicated to Shiva, it's popularly called Kashmir Shaivism. Other names include Trika Shasana or Trika Shastra, both meaning "triad teaching," Svatantrya ("independence"), Spanda ("throb, quiver, vibration"), and Trika (triad). This last name has been interpreted in different ways. It can, for example, refer to a mash-up of three ways of looking at Reality, monism (*abheda*, "unbroken") and dualism (*bheda*, "broken"), and nondual-cum-dual (*bheda abheda*), or difference-in-identity, or to the system's three major players, Shiva, Shakti, and Anu ("atom") or Nara ("person")—that is, the individual follower. In the grand scheme of things, we're another inseparable aspect of the divine. The only thing that keeps us from reuniting with true Self is our stubborn insistence that we're individuals—a mistaken belief that inevitably leads to all sorts of difficulty in life, which in time will instigate the search for the true Self.

The three universes of monism, dualism, and triadism provide an interesting contrast. The monist universe is a superimposition. It's often compared to a misapprehension, seeing what appears to us as a snake until we take a closer look and discover it's a rope. It only has a relative reality, and once Atman realizes itself, the snake-universe is seen for what it is, rope-Brahman. Patanjali's universe is by itself an insentient process with no innate value of its own, its entire existence serving only to "entertain and liberate" the Self.[17] Upon liberation, when that Self is seen for what it truly is, the universe's "purpose is fulfilled,"[18] and that little bit of cherished matter which we all along mistakenly believed to be "me" is abandoned for forever and resolved back into the Universal matrix.

The Trika Universe, in contrast, is the *lila* of the goddess, a word defined as "play, sport, diversion, amusement, pastime." This suggests the enormous gap that exists between us humans, who often have so much difficulty managing a single life of our own, and the deity, to whom the entire universe is just "child's play" and the "ease or facility in doing anything," two further meanings of lila. In Triadism, the goddess is both the material and the efficient cause of the universe; in other words, she creates everything that exists out of her own substance, her own body, which is then suffused with Shiva consciousness. The universe is here completely real and aware, with astounding "grace, charm, beauty," yet more meanings for lila.

We read over and over again in Hatha texts how this or that exercise "destroys" disease, old age, and death. Patanjali yogis and Advaitins want to escape from the suffering they believe accompanies an attachment to matter. Trika yogis though want "embodied liberation" (*jivanmukti*, see p. 182), that is, to both achieve Self-liberation and live far beyond the normal span of years so they can continue to enjoy the loveliness of our world.

3

THE YOGA WORLD
BY THE NUMBERS

All this circuit of the earth, encompassed by garlands of lands
and forests and mountains and cities and oceans, and encircled
by the Lokaloka mountains, extends, is comprehended, in the
midst of the Egg of Brahma.

Vyasa commenting on *Yoga Sutra* 3.26

TWO EGGS (*ANDA*): THE BALL EGG (*PINDA ANDA*) AND THE BRAHMA EGG (*BRAHMA ANDA*)

In oneself lies the whole world, and if you know how to look
and learn, then the door is there and the key is in your hand.
Nobody on earth can give you either that key or the door to
open, except yourself.

Jiddu Krishnamurti, *You Are the World*

I have a book in my library, just over 750 pages in length, titled *The
Dictionary of Imaginary Places*. All the places we might expect to be included are there—Middle Earth, Wonderland, Never-Never Land, Nar-
nia, Lilliput, Oz—the two authors did a magnificent piece of work. Yet
they overlooked one place, possibly because neither is a yoga student or

possibly because the place isn't considered "imaginary." This is the world of the Brahma egg (*brahma anda*), named after Brahma, the creator deity of the Hindu triple form (*trimurti*), or trinity.

This egg is described in several of the texts belonging to the genre of Indian literature known as the Puranas, or "ancient tales." If you would like to read this story for yourself, here are four Puranas you can look in, all available online in English: *Vishnu Purana*, book 2, chapter 2; *Markendaya Purana*, cantos 54–55; *Brahma Purana* chapters 16–21; *Linga Purana* chapters 46–53.

We also find this world detailed in a commentary by Vyasa to *Yoga Sutra* 3.26, a sutra that tells us how to access the egg by meditating on the "sun," though it's not clear if Patanjali means our system's star or a subtle structure in the body. Whichever it is, it's not really important to us. For our purposes, we'll go with Vyasa's commentary, which happens to be the longest among his 40 or so commentaries to the sutras of the supernormal powers in YS 3.

The first thing we might notice about this world is that it's shaped like an enormous disk. On it are seven concentric islands, each separated from the one surrounding it by a sea, seven in all, only one of which is filled with salt water. The others have sugarcane juice, wine, butter, curd, cream, and milk. Anyone for a nice day at the beach sipping a glass of seawater?

At the center of these seven islands, like the bull's-eye of a target, is the "king of mountains," Mount Meru. To call it a mountain doesn't quite do it justice, though. Its four slopes are silver, emerald, crystal, and gold; its elevation is estimated at 84,000 yojanas. There's some disagreement among the various sources about the length of a yojana in miles; the low-end estimation is four miles and the high, eight. It hardly matters, since Meru is at least 336,000 miles high, which means if it were one of Earth's mountains, we could climb it all the way to the moon and beyond. By comparison, our tallest mountain, Chomolungma—otherwise known as Everest—is just under five and a half miles high.

The Brahma egg's population is diverse, to say the least. There are gods and demigods of all kinds; virtuous humans after they've died; demons, ghosts, imps, ogres, and nymphs; and even a group of beings that defy categories—the Kimpurushas: literally, "What sort of person?" Some of the gods live for a thousand kalpas, which is more than four trillion years, slightly more than 285 times longer than the estimated 14-billion-year life of our universe. They've mastered the elements, there's "no impediment to their thinking" and so they're essentially omniscient, and they feed on contemplation. The farthest reaches of this world are rimmed by the Lokaloka Mountains, 500 million yojanas (or at least two billion miles) in extent. And all of this? It's ultimately just a "minute fragment of the primary-cause, like a firefly in the sky."

Now the Brahma egg isn't the only egg of its kind. There's a second one, called the ball egg (*pinda anda*), that's supposed to be an exact recreation of its humongous sibling, only this one's our body. How do the yogis explain the existence of the two eggs? One possibility is offered by Kshemaraja, the Tantric philosopher. He speculated that the world itself is Shiva's body, and each of us, like Shiva, "has the body of the entire universe in a contracted form even as the fig tree is in a contracted form in its seed."[1]

The idea of body-as-world is very old in India. The earliest reference I found is in the *Atharva Veda*, usually dated sometime between 1200 to 1000 BCE. Here we're introduced to one of the mysterious Vratyas (from *vrata*, "religious vow"), a group of wandering mendicants about which not much is known. Scholars have called them ascetics, mystics, or precursors of the yogis, and what distinguished them was the ram skin slung over each shoulder—one light-colored, one dark. The AV compares the Vratya's vital breaths to features of the world, to the Earth, the waters, domesticated and other animals, to the skies, constellations, the sun and moon, and heaven.

Of that Vratya.
The right eye is the Sun and the left eye is the Moon.
His right ear is Agni and his left ear is Pavamana.
Day and Night are his nostrils. Diti and Aditi are his
    head and skull.

By day the Vratya is turned westward, by night
    he is turned eastward.
Worship to the Vratya![2]

If we jump ahead at least 2,000 years, we'll find a beautifully composed, early example of the body-as-world in third chapter of the *Siddha
Siddhanta Paddati* (SSP), a text attributed to the guru Goraksha. The
seven islands are situated in places like the bones, hair, and fingernails,
the seven oceans in the bodily fluids, and rivers flow through the subtle
energy channels (*nadis*). Deities and other divine or malignant beings
reside in the pores of the skin or the prana. In one especially striking
passage, it's said that "many clouds inhabit the tears. Infinite numbers of
siddhas [i.e., sages] inhabit the luminosity of the intellect. The moon and
sun dwell in the pair of the eyes."[3]

And what about Meru? Have you ever heard of the Meru *danda*, the
"staff of Meru"? That's the name with which the yogis honor our spine,
homologizing it with the king of mountains. Why a staff? A staff is a
yogi's support as he makes his way across the length and breadth of India
on his endless pilgrimage; in the same way, our spine is our central support as we make our way through the pilgrimage of our lives. The chapter concludes with a very positive affirmation. We're told the "Supreme
Lord of the Universe, the Supreme Soul, exists in every individual body
in the form of pure consciousness of indivisible nature."[4]

THREE STRANDS (*GUNA*):
TAMAS, RAJAS, SATTVA

The seen (i.e., Nature) has the character of brightness, activity,
and inertia (i.e., resistance to motion).

Yoga Sutra 2.18

Patanjali's world is made of *prakriti*, the "original or primary substance."
Prakriti in turn is composed of three strands (*guna*), named *tamas* (inertia), *rajas* (energy), and *sattva* (light), which are sometimes pictured
as wound around each other like the fibers of a rope. Three is the min-

imum number of components needed to account for the world's diversity. If there were just one strand, everything would be made of the same stuff and there would be no diversity. If there were two strands, there are two possibilities: they would cancel each other out, or one would dominate and bury the other. In either case, again, no diversity. With three strands the game is on, and neither can they cancel nor can one dominate the others.

In the beginning, before there was a world, the strands coexisted in perfect equilibrium, and they would have remained so for all eternity had not the Self wandered by. Here we encounter two of the unsolved mysteries of Patanjali Yoga. The first is: why?

Why does the Self involve itself in matter at all? After all, as soon as it does, its only purpose is to find a way to separate itself again. It seems like it could have saved itself a lot of trouble simply by avoiding the involvement. Patanjali Yoga is mum on this question, or it shrugs its shoulders and says, that's the way it's always been.

The second mystery concerns the relationship between the two existents. The Self is unchanging but sentient, though that sentience is of nothing in particular, since the Self has no organs with which it could be sentient of something. Matter, conversely, is always changing but doesn't know it is because it's completely insentient. Each then has the quality the other lacks to complete itself, and it seems like a marriage made in yoga heaven. But in Patanjali's curious world, no contact between the two principals is possible; they're forever radically separate. And yet, still, nevertheless, just the Self's nearness to matter is enough to disturb the strands' harmony and kick-start the world process.

The image of a magnet and iron filings is sometimes used to explain what happens. The former can act on the latter just by being nearby; that is, the magnet can influence the filings at a distance. We can say there's a magnetic sympathy between the two, as it's in the nature of the magnet to attract the filings and in the nature of the filings to be attracted by the magnet. But we're cautioned not to think of this event as creation per se, since the Self doesn't act purposefully on matter. It appears that in Patanjali Yoga, the world just happens.

It's also tempting to think of the three strands as distinct, and to some extent they are, since they often oppose each other. But at the same time, they're intimately dependent on each other and can't ever be completely split apart. As the *Samkhya Karika* notes, they "mutually and successively dominate, support, and interact with one another."[5] Like Brahma, Vishnu, and Shiva—the Big Three of the Hindu trinity—the gunas form a one-for-all and all-for-one trio.

Each guna manifests specific qualities, both physical or objective and, because human consciousness is material, psychological or subjective (see p. 30). Tamas supplies things with heaviness and inertia or resistance to change. Rajas is the energy that moves things, that powers change. Sattva, which is technically on the opposite end of the spectrum from tamas, can be defined as lightness, which has two meanings (actually three, but one doesn't concern us): in the sense of illumination and in the sense of weightlessness. Something that's lightweight and/or brightens things up is sattvic. Everything material—which is to say, everything that exists—is composed of varying proportions of the three gunas, including all of us.

In that regard, the dictionary tells us that tamas is the "basis of all lack of feeling, dullness, ruthlessness, insensibility . . . , mental gloom, ignorance, error, and illusion." There's quite a bit more, but I think you get the picture: this is what your brain is like on tamas.

Rajas hardly fares better. This guna obscures our view, not only of the world, but of ourself. It drives our "desires, likes and dislikes, competition" and compels us to "strive for the goods of life, regardless of the needs and sufferings of others."

The nature of sattva contrasts sharply with its two mates: "living or sentient being, character, existence, reality, being, spiritual essence, magnanimity, consciousness, true essence, courage, quality of purity or goodness, good sense, goodness, strength of character, wisdom, resolution, life." No wonder Patanjali urges us to cultivate purity (*shauca*), which in turn purifies "*sattva*, gladness (*saumanasya*), one-pointedness, mastery of the sense organs (*indriya*), and the capacity for seeing the Self (*atman*)."[6]

Here's the way Patanjali Yoga is able to cross the seemingly unbridgeable gulf its dualistic worldview opens between purusha and prakriti. Though the existent is itself and nothing else, when consciousness is purged of as much tamas and rajas as possible, leaving a predominance of sattva, then it's as close to the Self as prakriti can ever get. The yogi can then experience what it might be like to finally be free of their prakriti and emerge as the true Self.

Though I can certainly understand the appeal of a sattvic consciousness, it seems to me that we can never be completely free of tamas and rajas no matter how hard and how long we metaphorically scrub at them. As long as we're embodied, then all three gunas must of necessity be part of and in operation in our lives.

But still, as a person who stubbornly clings to life, I have to wonder what would happen if we went in the opposite direction. If instead of tipping the scale to favor sattva, we return to the source before the world was born, when each of the gunas perfectly balanced the other two. Would we then be able to appreciate the solidity of tamas in counterpoint to the airiness of sattva, imbued with the passion of rajas? Would that open us to the Self without having to abandon the world?

FOUR AGES (*YUGA*)

Mortals at first a blissful Earth enjoy'd
With ills untainted, nor with cares annoy'd;
To them the world was no laborious stage,
Nor fear'd they then the miseries of age.
Hesiod, *Works and Days* (ca. 700 BCE)

"Official science teaches that man appeared on the earth in an imperfect state, from which he has since been gradually, though continually raising himself."[7] So writes Sir John Woodroffe, under the pseudonym Arthur Avalon, expressing a view that's likely shared by most Westerners in the twenty-first century. As humans, our favored story goes, we started out in a rather "imperfect state," as Woodroffe kindly frames it. Then after a treacherous evolutionary journey—though gradual, nevertheless continual—over who knows how many hundreds of thousands of years, we "raised" ourselves in some indefinite way at least somewhat out of our original condition. The implication is that this effort is still in process and one day it might be possible to raise ourselves if not to perfection, then to a state very close to it. Woodroffe continues: "Such teaching is, however, in conflict with the traditions of all peoples."[8] Oh.

The lines from the Greek poet Hesiod aren't singing presciently about modern humans, instead they're recalling what people were like when we first appeared on the Earth, our Golden Age, when people were exactly who we—with our conflicted official scientific view—want to be like in the future. Sadly this age came to an end, as humans fell away from their original perfection and became increasingly flawed, physically, psychologically, and spiritually. Then in slow succession, we descended through ages named after metals of decreasing value: silver, bronze, and now to iron. (Hesiod included a fifth age—the Heroic—between the bronze and iron, but typically yoga's classical view had four ages.)

Traditional India also asserts, along with Hesiod, that as far as cosmic history goes we don't *end* in perfection, we *begin* that way. Then, over a staggeringly long stretch of time, we slowly regress until we descend into an age of darkness, as if we slowly moved from Rivendell to Mordor. But no worries. Unlike Western time, which runs on a straight track from a fixed beginning to a final end, Indian time is cyclical. Every dark age is eventually succeeded by a new enlightened age, and the entire process repeats itself again and again, ad infinitum, which is to say, gradually but continually forever.

The basic unit of this regressive scheme is the *yuga*, four of which combine to make a great cycle or *maha yuga*. You probably noticed a rather familiar word in the last sentence. If we remove the *u* from *yuga* and replace it with an *o*, we get a word we all know quite well. In fact, *yoga* and *yuga* are related through their root *yuj*, "to yoke or join," though it's not clear how this meaning applies to a yuga. Where Hesiod's ages were named after metals, the yugas were individually named after four dice throws of decreasing luck, which seems odd until you know the backstory.

The Game of Dice and Naming the Four Yugas

Gambling, especially with dice, was an extremely popular pastime in India among all classes all the way back to Vedic times, at least 3,200 years ago. It was so popular, in fact, that even in the RV, Hinduism's holiest text, we find a poem famously known as the Gambler's Lament.[9] It was written in the first person to tell the sad tale of someone who was painfully addicted to gambling, complaining that dice are "armed with goads and driving-hooks, deceiving and tormenting, causing grievous woe." If the poet were alive today—and with reincarnation he may well be—he would most likely be a prime candidate for Gamblers Anonymous. He had apparently gambled away much or all of his wealth to the detriment of his homelife and marriage. "For the die's sake," he grieves, "mine own devoted wife I alienated," and what's worse, "her mother hates me" too. His advice to the rest of us is heartbreakingly poignant: "Play not with dice: no, cultivate thy corn-land. Enjoy the gain, and deem that wealth sufficient."

In Vedic times the dice were commonly fashioned from a kind of nut, brown in color, with only four pip surfaces instead of the six we're accustomed to today on our cube-shaped dice. Each side was named after the number of pips it displayed: the four-pip side was *krita*, the three-pip *treta*, the two-pip *dvapara*, and the one-pip *kali*. Scholars are unsure how the dice were used for gaming; however, they can say that krita, which also means "accomplished, proper, cultivated, good," was the winning throw. But if you threw kali, which also means "strife, discord, quarrel, contention, worst of a class or number of objects," you would surely have reason to sympathize with the *Rig Veda* gambler.

◂ ◂

Krita and *kali* are interesting words because they do triple duty: First, they name the number of pips on one side of a die. Second, in the context of the game of dice, they also comment on the expected reaction to the throw of that number: winning krita is good, while losing kali is worst of a class. And third, those comments also apply to the yugas they name. Krita Yuga, the Indian equivalent of Hesiod's Golden Age, is cultivated and accomplished. Kali Yuga, the Indian Iron Age, is the worst of the four yugas, and sometimes called the Age of Strife.

The two other words, *dvapara* and *treta*, are dicier. *Dvapara* also means "doubt, uncertainty," but since we don't know how the dice game to which this refers was played, we can't tell if those meanings had anything to say about a two-throw. Regardless, they do have some relation to Dvapara Yuga, in which "differences of opinion continually occurred among men . . . and a lack of firm resolve regarding the truth."[10] *Treta* is just along for the ride, its only meaning being "three."

Note that the order of the yugas and the numbers assigned to them are reversed, the earlier yuga is numbered four, and the latter is numbered one. Given the popularity of gambling, and knowing how well the definitions of krita and kali captured the zeitgeist—the spirit of the yugas to which they would be assigned—it's no surprise they rolled the dice and used their names.

▸ ▸ BEHIND THE NUMBERS

How Long Were the Yugas?

There are two basic time units to consider when dealing with the yugas, divine years and human years. One of the former equals 360 of the latter. I'm not sure why there are two time scales since they both measure the same thing. To avoid confusion, we'll just look at the human years.

The first yuga, Krita, was the longest of the four: its main time frame covered 1,440,000 years. As we regressed farther and farther away from our dharma, as our anxiety and perplexity increased, as we abandoned good works, each main yuga decreased 360,000 years from its predecessor. So Treta lasted 1,080,000 years, the Dvapara 720,000 years, and the Kali, the current age, is scheduled to last 360,000 years. But that's not all. Each yuga, much like every day in our lives, was preceded by its own "sunrise" and followed by a "sunset" called a *sandhya* (junction). Each sandhya equaled 10 percent of the yuga's main time frame. So for example, the two Krita sandhyas were each 144,000 years, which then means the full length of that yuga was 1,728,000 years. Accordingly then, the Treta totaled 1,296,000 years, the Dvapara 864,000 years, and the Kali, our current age, is scheduled to last 432,000 years. A maha yuga totals 4,320,000 years, and the cycles followed one after another like boxcars on a passing train, the caboose of which isn't in sight. (Note here, for future reference, that each of these totals is divisible by 108.)

The continued succession of the yugas—and the existence of the universe—depends on Brahma, the creator deity. We might expect that as a deity he would be eternal, but no: Brahma has a life span just as you or I do, though slightly longer. One day in his life, called a *kalpa*, equals 2,000 maha yugas, or 8,640,000,000 years. So one year of his life equals 3,110,400,000,000 years, and since he lives for 100 years, Brahma's full life span is 311,040,000,000,000 human years, that's 311 trillion 40 billion years. According to tradition—though we wonder who's doing the counting and how—Brahma has just passed the midpoint in his life, and so is 50 going on 51. That's the equivalent of about 155 trillion years, but not yet eligible for social security.

◄ ◄

So what were the people of the Krita Yuga like? The *Maha Nirvana Tantra* (MNT) has nothing but praise for them. Imagine everybody living strictly but willingly in accord with an extremely demanding moral code. We're told they were exceedingly powerful, courageous, strong and vigorous, wise and truthful, and of firm resolve. No one was selfish, thievish, malicious, foolish, envious, wrathful, gluttonous. They were all of "good heart and blissful mind," and they all attained final liberation.[11] It certainly didn't hurt that the land was amazingly fertile, the government well run, and the average life span was in the thousands of years.

How did it happen then that this idyllic world fell from grace and descended through the Treta and Dvapara Yugas into the Kali? Most scholars attribute it to a natural process of aging, something that afflicts both yugas and people.[12]

I won't go into the Treta and Dvapara Yugas in any detail, since it's the first and fourth yugas we're most curious about. Let's just recognize that as the centuries passed and the regressive behaviors became more prevalent and more inhuman, and after slightly less than 4,000,000 years, we find ourselves in the Kali Yuga.

Now what about the Kali Yuga? What does the MNT have to say about our age? By tradition the Kali begins right after the bloody conclusion of the great Indian civil war recounted in the MaB, an epic poem of gargantuan length, that provides the context for the BG. The traditional date for the war's end is February 18, 3102 BCE. When we add this number to the year in which I'm writing this, 2022, we find the MaB war ended 5,124 years ago. Then if we subtract that number from 432,000, we can project the end of the Kali Yuga to February 18 in the year 426,876. Be sure to circle that date on your calendar; you won't want to miss the closing ceremonies. Remember though, this will mark the end of the *current* maha yuga, not the end of everything—that's still a long way down the road.

It would be hard to exaggerate the differences between the Kali and the Krita; they're actually polar opposites. The MNT pulls no punches about the Kali people, which is to say, us. We're "gluttonous, cruel, heartless, harsh of speech, deceitful, mean, thievish, malicious, quarrelsome, greedy, impostors who think themselves wise, bent upon injury to the good," and the beat goes on. I've omitted the most egregious behaviors so as not to portray us as total and unredeemable beasts and dump us into a deep depression.[13] Does the MNT seem prescient to you? Is this how you'd describe the twenty-first century?

▸ ▸ YOGA BY THE NUMBERS

Four in Sanskrit

The Sanskrit word for four is *catur*. Four is the number of completion, perfection, and order, and we find it everywhere throughout the yoga tradition. There are four Vedas (*catur veda*)—the *Rig, Yajur, Sama*, and *Atharva*—at the very foundation of mainstream Hindu spirituality. There are four stages of life—unmarried student (*brahmacarin*), married householder (*grihastha*), forest dweller (*vanaprastha*) who lives an ascetic existence in the woods (*vana*), and mendicant (*samnyasin*, literally "laying aside, giving up, abandoning, renouncing"), who "abandons or resigns worldly affairs . . . and devotes himself to meditation." There are four goals in life (*purusha artha*, "human purpose")—*artha*, "substance, wealth, property"; *kama*, "pleasure, enjoyment"; *dharma*, "virtuous conduct"; and *moksha*, "emancipation, liberation."

Patanjali's YS has four chapters, and he knows a fourth state of breathing practice beyond inhaling, exhaling, and purposeful retention as a spontaneous stoppage of the breath called *caturtha*.[14] Vyasa, commenting on YS 2.15, compares Patanjali's system to the four aspects (*catur vyuha*) of a medical diagnosis and treatment—that is, disease, cause of disease, health, and remedy. For yoga the equivalent steps are *samsara*, the unending round of birth-death-rebirth which is the "disease"; the cause of *samsara*, which is Self-ignorance (*avidya*); the "cure" is release from *samsara* through Self-realization; and the means of release, yoga, is the remedy.

Like the YS, the VS is divided into four books, and then takes one step further by dividing each chapter into four parts. The first four sutras (*catuh sutri*) of the VS, composed in the second century BCE by Badarayana, are said to distill the essence of the entire teaching of Vedanta. The first sutra begins the inquiry into Brahman; the second defines it; the third singles out the source of our knowledge of Brahman; and the fourth "attempts to demonstrate the supreme value of the knowledge of Brahman."[15]

◂ ◂

4

SHIVA AND SHAKTI
BY THE NUMBERS

Philosophically speaking, Shiva is the unchanging Consciousness, and Shakti is its changing Power appearing as mind and matter. Shiva-Shakti is therefore Consciousness and its Power. This then is the doctrine of the dual aspects of the one Brahman. . . .

    Arthur Avalon (Sir John Woodroffe), *Shakti and Shakta*

Hindu deities often have more than the normal allotment of organs, limbs, or heads, a clear sign there's something special, or at least different, about them. Most people see the world well enough with two eyes, so a third eye might seem superfluous. But Shiva's third eye is mostly turned inward, away from the outer, mundane world. Its focus is figuratively but also quite literally on "in-sight," on the "in-tuitive" wisdom of the Self.

But watch out if he turns that eye around and looks out at the world: then it becomes a kind of flamethrower. Just ask Kama, the Hindu Cupid, who learned an important lesson when he mischievously drilled the meditating Shiva with one of his love-inducing arrows. Shiva, displaying all the restraint of a three-year-old rudely awakened from his nap, didn't appreciate being distracted. He turned toward Kama and

A great flame of fire sprang up from the third eye of the infuriated Śiva. That fire originating instantaneously from the eye in the middle of His forehead blazed with flames shooting up and resembling the fire of final dissolution in refulgence. After shooting up in the sky, it fell on the ground and rolled over the earth all round. Even before the gods had the time to say "Let him be forgiven, let him be excused" it reduced Kama to ashes.[1]

Sounds like Shiva needs to work a bit more diligently on his meditation practice.

▸ ▸ BEHIND THE NUMBERS

Why Do Hindu Gods Often Have More Than Two Arms?

A figure with three eyes, even though a deity, seems pretty strange to us here in the West, accustomed as we are to by-the-textbook Western anatomy. But the strangeness isn't limited to three eyes. When we look at drawings or photos of icons of Hindu deities, we might notice something else that's odd about them: many of them frequently have more than two arms. Why is that? The obvious answer is that it leaves no doubt they're not human, that there's something otherworldly and special about them. But it's not the arms alone that make them different.

We also notice their hands are often holding enough weapons to equip an army—axes, spears, swords, clubs, and much more—or random things—waterpots, feathers, flags, flowers, nets—or making symbolic gestures, called mudras ("seals," see p. 141). Unless we know something about Hindu iconography, the far-reaching meaning expressed by the figure and what its hands are holding or how they're shaped is lost on us or completely misunderstood.

It wasn't all that long ago that Ananda Coomaraswamy commented that certain writers, when "speaking of the many-armed images of Indian art, have treated this peculiarity as an unpardonable defect." He goes on to quote a critic who disparaged such images by opining they "have no pretensions to beauty, and are frequently hideous and grotesque."[2] Fortunately, with the growing popularity of yoga in the West, these misguided ideas are slowly disappearing.

We can sometimes tell something about a person's profession or hobby if they are pictured holding some implement or tool characteristic of that profession or hobby. For example, chances are a person holding a stethoscope is some sort of doctor, a small paintbrush and palette an artist, a Louisville Slugger a baseball enthusiast. The same goes for Hindu deities: what they're holding in their hands forcefully indicates to those in the know who they are and the areas and extent of their powers.

I made an extremely informal survey of books in my library with photos and drawings of Hindu deities (including the stunningly beautiful *Yoga: The Art of Transformation*), and can say with the unjustified confidence of the amateur sleuth that the most common number of arms is four, though eight, ten, and twelve arms crop up every now and then. The number four, as we see throughout this book, is highly significant in Indian culture and in yoga. It also represents the four yugas or ages of human history, the four castes of society, the four central aims and periods of our lives (*purusha artha*), the four Vedic samhitas, and the list goes on.

◄ ◄

As I mentioned, Shiva's three eyes represent the "light" of the world, with the understanding that there are two "lights" we need to see the world: the combined lights of sun, moon, and fire, which illuminates the outer world, and the light of consciousness, which illuminates the inner. Because he's both omniscient and omnipotent, the eyes also symbolize the times of past, present, and future and the forces needed to create, sustain, and reabsorb the world; that is, wisdom (*jnana*), desire or will (*iccha*), and action (*kriya*).

Shiva's three eyes have several names: *trilocana* (*locana*, "illuminate, brighten"), *trinetra* (*netra*, "guide," i.e., the eye as the "guiding organ"), *trinayana* (*nayana*, "pupil," and "leading, directing"), *tryaksha* (*aksha*, another name for "soul"), and *tryambaka* (*ambaka*, "eye"). Most of these words for eye can also be prefixed with *one* (*eka*) to emphasize the third eye alone: *ekanetra, ekalocana, ekanayana, ekaksha* all mean "one eye," referring of course to that one special eye.

The BG suggests it's also possible for each of us to develop a kind of third eye. Our third eye won't, of course, pop open in the middle of our forehead. But it helps us discern the difference between the "field" (*kshetra*) or universe and the "field-knower" (*kshetra jnayos*) or the Self, which liberates us from "material nature" so that we may realize the Supreme (*para*).[3] This eye goes by names like divine eye (*divya cakshus*), divine gaze (*diyva drishti*), and wisdom eye (*jnana cakshus* and *jnana netra*).

SHIVA AND HIS TRIDENT (*TRISHULA*), A THREE-PRONGED SPEAR

The trident (*trisul*) is . . . an ancient scepter of overlordship.
Wolf-Dieter Storl, *Shiva: The Wild God of Power and Ecstasy*

Another significant three associated with Shiva is the three prongs of his trident (*trishula, shula,* "spike, spear"), an emblem of his supremacy. The trident isn't his only weapon. He's also armed with a spear, an ax, a bow, and for good measure, a club topped with a human skull.

The prongs of the trident are associated with various threes: the three gunas of sattva, tamas, rajas; the three times of past, present, and future; Shiva's three aspects of creator, preserver, and reabsorber; the three main subtle arteries of ida, pingala, and sushumna; and the three-fold nature of Shiva/Shakti power—the power of will (*iccha shakti*), which decides to create the world with all its diversity; the power of knowledge (*jnana shakti*), which devises how to go about the creation; and the power of action (*kriya shakti*), which, based on desire and knowledge, brings the universe into being. The trident's shaft stands for the central axis around which the grand edifice will turn, while the two side prongs, when combined, form a crescent moon, a symbol of "rebirth and regeneration."[4]

It's common for people who admire a certain individual to try to imitate that person in appearance and behavior. Those yogis who revere Shiva are no exception, and many of them carry a trident in honor of their patron saint. Originally, it was made of animal horns, but after the invention of copper casting the horns were "replicated in the new metal alloy."[5] This accomplished two things: since copper is considered a solar metal, the trident now was closer symbolically to Shiva's; moreover, with metal prongs, it became a seriously lethal weapon.

Why did the yogi need a weapon? In the old days, wandering across the countryside, yogis occasionally needed to defend themselves against "wild animals, who were not so impressed by the ascetic's holiness as popular folk tales suggest."[6] Even today, a trident-wielding yogi presents an imposing figure, certainly encouraging any potential attacker to reconsider.

SHIVA AND HIS FIVE ACTIONS (*KRITYA*)

All inanimate life is believed to be ruled by the prime number 3 and its multiples by 2 and 3. Life, sensation, appears only when the number 5 becomes a component of the inner structure of things. The number 5 is associated with Shiva, the Progenitor, the source of life.

Alain Danielou, *The Gods of India*

It wouldn't be an exaggeration to call Shiva the Lord of Fives. Five, writes Stella Kramrisch, is the "sacred number of Shiva."[7] He has five aspects, or faces (*panca anana*), five actions (*panca kritya*), five cloaks (*panca kancuka*), five components (*panca kala*), and five powers (*panca shakti*). There are even five syllables (*panca akshara*) in his main mantra (NA-MA SHI-VAY-UH).

I bow to the divine who brings about emanation (*srishti*), re-absorption (*samhara*), concealment (*vilaya*), maintenance of the world (*sthiti*), who dispenses grace (*anugraha*), and who destroys the afflictions of those who have bowed down (to him).[8]

In considering Shiva's fives, we also have to digress and consider the Hindu triple form (*trimurti*). Shiva wasn't always in complete control of the functioning of the universe. Once upon a time, more than 2,000 years ago, that universe was overseen by a triumvirate consisting of Shiva and two other deities, Brahma and Vishnu. Brahma was the head of the creation department (*shrishti*, literally "letting go"). Vishnu saw to the maintenance of the universe's day-to-day workings (*sthiti*). And Shiva had the chore of bringing the current cycle to an end (*samhara*, "contraction, fetching back"), its matter to be recycled for the next go-round. At first glance, we might see these three as individual figures, each with a memorable name and distinguishing features; but in fact, as their collective name indicates, they're forms or manifestations by implication of Brahman, the "One Power of the universe." The third- or fourth-century BCE *Mandukya Upanishad* describes how they were "impelled" in turn by Brahman to go "on to differentiation"—Shiva, Brahma, and Vishnu in that order—each one a different persona of their source.[9]

▸ ▸ BEHIND THE NUMBERS

The Trimurti and the Trinity

A few scholars have raised the question: is there an equivalence between the trimurti and the Christian trinity of the Father, Son, and Holy Ghost? Several writers casually referred to the trimurti as the "Hindu trinity." But one writer squarely in the "definitely no" camp is the French author and confirmed traditionalist Rene Guenon. He insists the word *trinity* should not be applied to the trimurti, that properly it must be reserved exclusively for the Christian concept. The only resemblance between the two groups is that they both have three aspects of divinity, nothing more. Guenon concludes that it's "quite impossible to bring the three terms of one ternary into conformity with the three terms of the other."[10]

But another French author, Indologist Alain Danielou, believes otherwise. He claims the symbols associated with the trimurti aren't "altogether unconnected"[11] with those of the Christian trinity, though I must admit I wasn't entirely convinced by his argument. Because one of Shiva's main symbols is the *lingam*, that is, the penis, Danielou cast him in the part of the Progenitor, whom he equated with God the Father. Then because he descends to Earth in troubled times to save humanity from itself, Vishnu was cast as the Protector, and equated with the Son, whom certain segments of the population deem Christ. And finally, because Brahma balances Shiva and Vishnu, he was equated with the link between Father and Son, the Holy Ghost.

◂ ◂

When we enter the world of the Shaivites though, Shiva is the alpha god who assumes all three of the trimurti's functions. Along with these three, Shiva has two more that, just as the others form a coherent trio, make a related pair. The first is called concealment (*tirobhava*). Who or what is being concealed from whom or what? We could say that Shiva is concealing himself from himself, so that he can then go off in search of that hidden Self in and through the universe he's just brought into being.

Of course, his Self-limitation is recreated in his universe's creatures: us, and likely all those countless other beings we think are out there on other Earth-like planets. We then—some of us knowingly, many of us not (yet)—go off on our own quest, mimicking that of the Absolute, looking for that hidden part of ourselves. This has been the focus of yoga practice for more than 2,000 years: the question "Who am I?"

Over the years I've been teaching, one of the most difficult questions I'm occasionally asked is why, if the universe is Shiva's "sportive play,"[12] is there so much suffering, much of it seemingly random and/ or undeserved. To someone dealing with a serious or fatal illness, say, or born to extreme poverty, the world might not seem especially playful. The answer is that Shiva doesn't see the world as humans do. To us, there are good things about being alive, then again there are things that aren't good at all. But to Shiva it's all the same. In his quest to discover the Self he's purposely concealed from himself, Shiva must experience everything from the heights of ecstatic joy to the depths of abject misery. It's nothing personal.

But however miserable our lives may seem, it's reassuring to know that we're not condemned to that misery forever. The last of Shiva's actions is grace (*anugraha*, "favor, kindness, conferring benefits"). In order to receive this, we first have to feel the confinement of our Self-limitation, our concealment. Next we should relax and release the tight structures that bind us as isolated individuals to experience the infiniteness of our true nature. "Then a process of overflowing, of spilling over the walls of the boundaries occurs."[13]

‣ ‣ BEHIND THE NUMBERS

The Dance of Shiva and His Five Actions

There are certain traditional Hindu images that appear over and again in the modern yoga world. The OM sigil is probably the most ubiquitous, but following close behind are the images of the pudgy elephant-headed Ganesha, the heartrending monkey chief Hanuman, and the Lord of the Dance, Shiva Nataraj. I don't think it's well-known, however, that "his dancing limbs convey by their movements and symbols the fivefold action of creation, maintenance, dissolution, veiling-unveiling, and liberation."[14]

In his upper right hand Shiva holds an hourglass-shaped drum, the *dameru*. His insistent, rhythmic thrumming of this instrument generates the mystic primal sound that emits the universe, *shrishti*, which conveys "revelation, tradition, incantation, magic, and divine truth."[15] This is opposed by the upper left hand, its upturned palm shaped in what's called the half-moon mudra (*ardha candra mudra*). It holds a tongue of flame that will someday, at the end of its life cycle, melt the universe down. These two hands then are in a counterpoise that express the "ceaselessness of production against an insatiate appetite of extermination, Sound against Flame."[16]

Both of Shiva's lower hands are shaped into mudras. The lower right hand is shaped in the "have no fear" mudra (*abhaya mudra*), palm facing forward with upturned fingers, that reassures us of Shiva's vigilant protection, *sthiti*, "staying or remaining," the maintenance of life. The lower left hand reaches across Shiva's torso and points down at the uplifted left foot. This hand imitates the outstretched trunk-"hand" of an elephant (*gaja hasta mudra*), a reminder of Shiva's son Ganesha, the remover of obstacles. Appropriately, the raised foot stands for final release and the refuge of the soul.[17]

◂ ◂

SHIVA AND HIS FIVE CLOAKS (*KANCUKA*)

[These] are the attributes of consciousness when it is in its most expanded, unconditioned state . . . , omnipotence, omniscience, perfect completeness, freedom from natural law and eternality.

Mark Dyczkowski, *The Doctrine of Vibration:*
An Analysis of the Doctrines and Practices of Kashmiri Shaivism

In order to hide himself from himself, to then go in search of himself, Shiva covers himself in "five cloaks" (*kancuka*), purposely limiting the attributes listed in the epigraph. Although "cloak" is the usual rendering of *kancuka* into English, it's useful to remember that the word also means "disguise" and the "skin of a snake." The kancukas not only limit Shiva's powers, they limit ours as well, and disguise the Self so we identify with the limitations. Our goal then is to outgrow these limitations as a snake does its skin, and when we do, slough it off. These cloaks/disguises are as follows.

1. Knowledge (*vidya*) limits our capacity to know and creates a duality, the idea that we are separate from the world and others. Dyczkowski points out that though we're then ignorant of the universe's underlying unity, this doesn't mean our "knowledge of diversity is false." Our ignorance is a form of knowledge which, though "quite correct, is binding."[18]

2. *Kala* (with a long second *a*, pronounced kuh-LAH, best left untranslated) limits our agency or the power of our actions.

3. Desire (*raga*) limits the fullness (*purnatva*) or completeness of the Self and creates a hunger for the objects of the world. Though not mentioned directly here, the implication is that, just as with Patanjali's *kleshas*, raga is mated with its opposite number, aversion (*dvesha*). After all, we can desire to have something or we can desire to avoid something.

4. *Kala* (with a long first *a*, pronounced KAH-luh) limits time and brings in its wake past, present, future, and mortality.

5. Necessity (*niyati*) is a form of determinism that limits our freedom of space (*svatantraya*). Someone bound by niyati is called a *pashu*, which means a "tethered animal."

SHAKTI'S FIVEFOLD ASPECTS

Shakti dissolves within Shiva. Shiva dissolves within Kriya. Kriya is dissolved within Jnana. Jnana dissolves within Iccha. The fire of the Supreme Shakti is where Iccha Shakti is dissolved.

Kaula Jnana Nirnaya 2.6

We shouldn't be surprised if Shakti has her own stable of fives to mirror those of Shiva. Two are found in the SSP, traditionally ascribed to Gorakshanath, though dated by scholars in the eighteenth century, hundreds of years after the life of the semilegendary guru.

▸ ▸ BEHIND THE NUMBERS

Two Meanings of Shakti

Literally, the definition of the word *shakti* gives a pretty good idea of what this deity is all about: "power, ability, strength, effort, energy, capability."

Figuratively, she's called Shakti because she's "dear to a hundred (shata) crores of the great divine Yogini deities, and because she grants quick liberation."[19] (Crore = 10,000,000, 100 crore = 1,000,000,000.)

◂ ◂

In the fourth chapter she's credited as being the substratum (*adhara*) of all bodies (*pinda*), including presumably the body of the universe. It's said she's "eternally awake" and the "root of cause, effect and doing," and for these reasons she's called the "supporting power" (*adhara Shakti*). With her fivefold form (*pancadha*), her qualities are illumination, existence or being, I-consciousness (*ahanta*), quivering (*sphurana*) or throbbing (*sphur*) as our life force (*prana*), and comprehension of all this in a state of purity, wisdom, and self-luminosity.[20]

In the first chapter of the SSP we find a very detailed description of the five-stage unfolding of the universe, which would give any modern-day cosmologist a run for their money. Each stage has five qualities, which trace the gradual separation of the power (Shakti) from the power holder (Shiva) through which the universe comes into manifestation. We could also compare it to the development of each of us from birth, when there's no sense of a separate Self or individual power, to maturity and the realization of ourselves as a stand-alone person with a wide range of expressive possibilities.

In ethereal, the process begins with Shiva-Shakti in complete integration, with no sense at all of difference between them. Shakti's qualities at this stage are a presence in the Self, purity, self-luminosity, and a "perfectly calm and tranquil" rest "in the bosom of Shiva."[21] At this first stage Shiva is Shakti and Shakti is Shiva.

At the second stage, Shakti begins to stir, but only slightly. She begins to awaken to her power to create the universe in all its staggering diversity, though she's still enwrapped in Shiva. The words used to describe the qualities of the third stage all derive from *sphura*, "quiver, throb," as Shakti now begins a serious push for external manifestation. This could almost describe the Big Bang: "flashing consciousness, emanation, expansion, bursting, and creative pulsation." In the fourth stage Shakti grows increasingly conscious of herself as separate from Shiva, though as yet there's no sense of duality and she has revealed a conviction or "fullness of self-knowledge" (*nishcaya*), which is also changeless (*nirvikalpata*). When the fifth and final unfoldment arrives, Shakti emerges as a "distinct Psychic Power"[22] and is known as kundalini shakti. Her qualities are completeness (*purnata*), reflectiveness (*pratibimbata*), which means she acts as a mirror in which Shiva can see himself "reflected in an infinite variety of forms," and an "infinite capability"[23] to create from within herself the various orders of existence, which she then also sustains and regulates.

Now as the power that manifests the universe, Shakti has five aspects.

1. *Cit Shakti*, the "power" of "pure consciousness" (*cit*), which fills Shiva with wonder and ananda, "pure happiness," bliss. Such bliss is the nature of the Self, so for Shiva-Shakti joy isn't "caused by any exterior thing as is the case with the bound individual." Shiva-Shakti is "made of joy, as it were . . . bliss constitutes the Self."

2. Since bliss also implies freedom, ananda-Shakti is defined as *svatantrya*, "freedom."[24]

3. The bliss encourages *iccha*, "the desire or will to create," its first spark (*camatkara*, "astonishment, festive turbulence"). This desire, remember, isn't like the average person's desire to create, in which we need to make an effort. Iccha "arises spontaneously and effortlessly."[25]

4. This desire can't be realized without *jnana*, the mental picture, like a blueprint, of what to create and how to create it.

5. Finally the external construction (*kriya*) of the universe begins.

Just as Shiva's five actions are divided three and two, so Shakti's aspects of iccha, jnana, and kriya make a trio and are often considered the principal powers, while cit and ananda are a duo.

▸ ▸ BEHIND THE NUMBERS

Five in Sanskrit

The Sanskrit word for five is *pancan* (in compounds prefixing other words, *panca*, pronounced pun-chuh). In the Sanskrit dictionary, *panca* also means "to spread out the hand with its five fingers." Pentads (the word is an offspring of *panca*) make an impressive showing in the yoga tradition. I think it's safe to say that this is due, at least in part, to the influence of our hands with their five fingers, which we can use to "think with" and "count on." To tote up all the pentads in the tradition using our digits like a child, we'd need all our fingers and toes, and maybe those of a few friends as well.

The VS recommends meditating on the "five deities": the three making up the *trimurti* (Brahma, the creator; Vishnu, the preserver; and Rudra, the "recycler"); the "great principle" (*mahat tattva*), the first appearance of consciousness in the universe (the macrocosmic equivalent to the microcosmic of the individual's intellect or buddhi); and the *avyakta*, the "primary germ of nature" from which the material world develops.[26]

Not to be outdone, there are also five female deities, the feminine aspects of Vishnu. They are:

- Durga, the "root and root cause of everything," eternal, all-powerful, the upholder of truth, who brings happiness, welfare, and salvation to her devotees.
- Radha, who presides over the five breaths (*pranas*), eternal and formless, "beyond attributes, unattached and detached," and so invisible to the naked eye. It's said that Brahma performed austerities (*tapas*) for 600 centuries just to catch a glimpse of her lotus feet, but failed.
- Lakshmi, the "universal soul," the personification of compassion, welfare, peace and goodness, forever sympathetic and kind to her devotees.
- Sarasvati, also a form of the universal soul, the goddess of intellect, reason and logic, poetical skill and language. Without her, humans couldn't speak.
- Savitri, the essence of truth, existence, and supreme bliss, granting salvation, purifying the world with the touch of her feet.[27]

The *Brahma Vidya Upanishad* (BVU) counts five *atmans* that divinize the physical body. Brahman sits in the heart, Vishnu in the throat, Rudra (Shiva) in the palate, Maheshvara ("great lord") in the forehead, and Sada Shiva (*sada*, "eternal") at the tip of the nose, the "supreme seat," which transcends or is "beyond the body" (*dehatita*).[28] Our heart has five channels or doors, each guarded by a different deity and each leading us to the Absolute. Our Self is wrapped in five sheaths (*kosha*), much like Shiva is wrapped in five cloaks, though for much different reasons.

Our world is composed of two related pentads of traditional elements: the gross Earth, Water, Fire, Air, and Ether and their subtle counterparts. These elements—typically combined with their symbols, mystic syllables (*panca varna, ya, ra, la, va, ha*), and reigning deities—are then concentrated in areas of the body, such as the heart or crown, and meditated upon, often for five *ghatikas* or two hours.[29] As with all such practices, success in each area generates a specific power in some way related to the element and the body focus: concentrate on the air element between the eyebrows for two hours to "bring about the ability to move through space."[30] Breaking down the "doorway to liberation" is usually the jackpot in all these meditations.

We interact with the world and other people through five knowing (*jnana indriya*) and five action (*karma indriya*) organs. The former include the eyes (*cakshus*), ears (*shrotra*), nose (*ghrana*), tongue (*rasa*), and skin (*tvac*). The latter are the voice (*vak*), hands (*pani*), feet (*pada*), anus (*paya*), and generative organ (*upastha*). The word *indriya* means "fit for or belonging or agreeable to Indra; a companion of Indra; power, force, the quality which belongs especially to the mighty Indra." This means that our organs are ultimately in the service of Brahman, who uses them, through us, to explore the world it created.

We have five "fires" burning in our subtle body, but don't be concerned about them spreading through our interior world; they're slow-burning and well contained. The first is the fire of time (*kala agni*), the lowest of the five located in the base cakra (*muladhara*). In succession then are the submarine fire (*vadaba*) burning in our bones, Earthy fire (*parthiva*) in our stomach, the fire in the midethereal region (throat? heart?) that looks like lightning and has the character of the interior of the atman. Finally the fire with the form of the Sun (*suryarupa*) is burning in our navel.

That intelligent yogi who conceives of these five fires by means of his intellect, whatever is eaten and drunk by him, partakes of the nature of a sacrificial offering alone. There is no doubt about it.[31]

It seems too that Patanjali was a fan of fives: there are five fluctuations (*vritti*) of consciousness that need stilling (*nirodha*), five restraints (*yama*) and five observances (*niyama*, see p. 108), five afflictions (*klesha*, see p. 119), and five stages of consciousness (*citta bhumi*, see p. 117), though technically this pentad is courtesy of Patanjali's first commentator Vyasa.

These are just a few of the pentads in the yoga tradition. There's no doubt here that five is a number to hold in awe, because as we'll see, it's built right into the fabric of the universe.

◄ ◄

5

SUBTLE BODY
BY THE NUMBERS

Psychologically, this ignorance of Brahman is marked by the superimposition (*adhyasa*) of what are technically called "sheathes"
(*kosas*) "over" . . . the underlying reality of Brahman-Atman, so
that man identifies himself with these *kosas* and thus apparently
(i.e., not actually) obscures his real identity with the Absolute.

Ken Wilber, *The Spectrum of Consciousness*

When we go out for the day, what's the one thing we always do before
stepping out the door? The answer I'm looking for—and I hope you
agree—is to put on clothes. Depending on the season of the year and
the weather outside, we might have just one or two layers if the day is
warm, three or four if it's cool or cold. Now the Self, when it enters
embodied life, does something similar. It wraps itself in a series of what
are called sheaths (*kosha*)—five in all—that decrease in density from
the outer to the core.

They're often depicted, Lama Govinda writes, as "separate layers,
which one after another crystallize around a solid nucleus"; the image
that comes to mind is the layers of an onion. For example, Ken Wilber, in the book from which the chapter epigraph is taken, says exactly
that, describing the outer koshas as the skin of the onion. This, the lama

contends, is inaccurate; instead, their nature is of "mutually penetrating forms of energy" from the subtlest to the densest, so that the former sheaths "penetrate, and thus contain" the latter.[1]

‣ ‣ BEHIND THE NUMBERS

Three Bodies (Sharira)

Our universe is divided into three levels, which correspond to levels of the body (although there are actually four levels if we count the Self). These are the gross body (*sthula sharira*), the subtle body (*sukshma sharira*), also known as the sign body (*linga sharira*), and the causal body (*karana sharira*). Each of these bodies is enjoyed by a different self, named *vishva* ("intellect"), *tejasa* ("power"), and *prajna* ("wisdom"), respectively. The five sheaths are then distributed among these three bodies.

◂ ◂

The outermost sheath, what we call the physical body, the yogis call the "sheath made of food" (*anna maya kosha*). It's called this, as Shankara explains, because "food made its birth possible; on food it lives; without food it must die."[2] This sheath is also known as the *sthula sharira*, the "tangible" or "gross" body, which is our flesh and blood vehicle. It's composed of six physical sheaths of skin (*tvac*), blood (*rakta*), flesh (*mamsa*), fat (*medas*), marrow (*majjan*), and bone (*asthi*), and the five traditional elements.

The next three sheaths, of increasing subtlety, make up the sukshma sharira, the "subtle body." The outermost of the three is called the "sheath made of vital energy" (*prana maya kosha*), that is, the 10 prana vayus (see p. 67). The next deeper sheath is the "sheath made of mind" (*manas maya kosha*). Because it includes and oversees the five organs of perception, it's usually thought of as the sixth sense. The third and deepest subtle body sheath is the "sheath made of intellect" (*vijnana maya kosha*), which works in tandem with the manas kosha. Manas receives information about the outside world through the senses, organizes it, then kicks it upstairs to the vijnana kosha. The vijnana decides on an appropriate response, then hands it back down to manas for execution. This, I hasten to add—as I'm sure you're already aware—is the ideal. Gathering, organizing, and relaying information can be faulty or misleading, and if it is, responses can be inappropriate or just plain wrong, even destructive.

The subtlest of the five sheaths is the "sheath made of bliss" (*ananda maya kosha*), the equivalent of the causal body (*karana sharira*). According to Shankara's dour assessment, this bliss isn't what we think it is; it's not the spontaneous joy we feel when approaching the Self. Rather it's just another "creation of our ignorance," which never comes to any good.[3] Here we're reminded that in this teacher's school of yoga there's only one desire that passes muster, and that's *mumukshu*, the desire for liberation. All other desires are a trap. There's a bit of controversy surrounding this sheath, which is whether or not it's the same as the Self. Most sources, including Shankara, say it isn't.

So now that the Self is covered in these sheaths, what do we do about it? We start with the familiar premise that because of Self-ignorance, we mistakenly identify exclusively with the five sheaths, that is, the material body. As we know, this misidentification of believing the body rather than the Self is the true Self is said to be the source of unremitting existential sorrow (*duhkha*). Here we have another map with which we can burrow down through the sheaths and find the cave hiding the Self.

This leads to a meditation called the "discrimination of the five sheaths" (*kosha pancaka viveka*), which is essentially a process of elimination. We take each sheath in turn beginning with the anna kosha and, pondering all the reasons it can't be the Self, gradually release our identification with each until nothing's left but the Self.

The *Pancadashi* provides a sort of meditation guide, explaining the reasons why each sheath can't be the Self. To simplify, the anna kosha can't be the Self because "it does not exist either before birth or after death";[4] in other words, it's not eternal as a Self would be. The prana vayus are scratched because they're "devoid of consciousness."[5] The manas sheath has desires, is "moved by pleasure and pain," and is subject to "delusions."

Worst of all, it's "fickle."[6] We already know how this school feels about desire. The intellect sheath is "changeable,"[7] and the bliss sheath is "temporal and impermanent,"[8] all very un-Self-like qualities.

10 ENERGY CHANNELS (*NADI*)

If they [i.e., the nadis] were revealed to the eye the body would present the appearance of a highly complicated chart of ocean currents.

Arthur Avalon (Sir John Woodroffe), *Shakti and Shakta*

Our bodies, as I'm sure you know, are crisscrossed from head to foot with veins and arteries that circulate blood toward and away from the heart. In Sanskrit, these channels are called *nadis*, though we need to qualify them as "coarse." That's because we also have a network of subtle nadis (called the *nadi cakra*, the "wheel of nadis") that circulate vital energy (*prana*) through the body. This network originates from an egg-shaped bulb (*kanda*) located either at the base of the spine or in the middle of the body in the vicinity of the navel.

▸ ▸ BEHIND THE NUMBERS

How Many Nadis Are There Altogether?

Yoga by the numbers isn't always tidy; sometimes the given numbers don't match. We see this when it comes to our body's energy channels. Most texts set the number at 72,000, of which, according to the *Yoga Cudamani Upanishad* (YCU), "seventy-two are specifically mentioned as important"[9] (though I've never been able to find a text that lists these 72). Now much like the number 84 (see p. 140), number 72 (and 72,000) isn't to be taken literally. Joseph Campbell writes that it's a number of "mythic magnitude, related to a science rather of a symbolic than of a strictly factual order."[10] It could, I suppose, be counted as a member of the 18 family (see p. 150), since that number multiplied by the number of completion—four—equals 72.

There are other texts, though, in which the nadis are numbered at three-and-a-half lakh, which equal 350,000. How can anyone accurately count that many subtle channels that snake over and around each other to every nook and cranny of our body? The answer is: no one can; this number, like all outsized numbers in yoga, is meant to awe and inspire.

To complicate things even further, I ran across a reference to "four-times-twenty thousand" nadis, or 80,000, in the *Tejo Bindu Upanishad* (TBU). Then, fewer than 10 verses on, the same text says the nadis are "seventy-two thousand in number," each with branches reaching out in all directions so they "cannot at all be counted."[11] It seems like the best way to think of the nadis is that they're countless.

◂ ◂

Just as the overwhelming multitude of asanas are whittled down to a more human scale (see p. 137), the 72,000 nadis are first reduced to 72, and then to 10. There are a couple with rather odd names, unless you think naming subtle channels odd in general. These are Elephant Tongue (*hasti jihva*) and Plenteously Misty (*alambusa*, Feuerstein's rendering). Then we have nadis appealingly named Nourishing (*pusha*), Splendid (*yashasvini*), New Moon (*kuhu*), Mother-of-Pearl (*shankhini*), and *ghandari*. This last name may not ring a bell unless you've read the MaB or the BG. Ghandari is the wife of the blind king Dhritarashtra and the mother of 100 sons along with one daughter.

Finally, the remaining three of the 10 nadis singled out as the most important are Comfort (*ida*), Reddish-Brown or Tawny (*pingala*), and Very Gracious (*sushumna*). This last one is credited as the most important of the 72,000, as it connects the base cakra, where the mysterious Kundalini slumbers, with the crown center. It's through this nadi that the awakened power will climb to its fulfillment in the *sahasrara cakra*, the thousand-spoked wheel at the crown.

We might imagine that the teaching about prana is unique to India, but in fact there are lots of traditional cultures that posit the existence of such a life force. The Chinese, for example, call it *chi* (also spelled *qi*), the Japanese call it *ki*, the Kung bushmen of Namibia call it "boiling energy." Actually, the old and widespread belief in a universal life energy has a name: vitalism. According to my dictionary, vitalism holds that "life processes arise from or contain a nonmaterial vital principle and cannot be explained entirely as physical and chemical phenomena." As loyal and trusting yoga students, we tend to accept without question what our teachers and the yoga tradition have to say about prana, not to mention other aspects of the subtle body, like the nadis and cakras.

Modern science, however, takes nothing for granted, and over the past 100 years or so has examined the world around us very carefully for some hint of this energy and found . . . well, nothing. Of course, we could say that science's instruments are incapable of measuring subtle energy and that what our scientist friends need to do is sit down and attend to their breathing as diligently as they monitor their instruments. This isn't likely to sway many of the nonbelievers; if it can't be measured, they'll insist, then it likely doesn't exist, and anyway, our life processes can be explained quite nicely without any recourse to a concept like vital energy.

Despite the discouraging response from the scientists, the modern West has its share of life force proponents, most of whom are considered rather odd ducks. We can take the nineteenth-century Baron Carl von Reichenbach of Germany as an example: A trained chemist who discovered kerosene, he claimed he'd found what he called the "Odic force" (apparently named after the Norse god Odin) that pervades the universe and keeps all its parts glued together. Then there's psychoanalyst Wilhelm Reich, who discovered what he called "orgone energy" in the 1930s, which he believed was nature's creative force. Reich was sent to prison in 1956 for what the Food and Drug Administration claimed was the illegal interstate shipment of his telephone-booth size "orgone accumulators," where he died the following year.

Comfort and Tawny, along with Very Gracious, make up the Big Three of the nadis, like the trimurti makes up the Big Three of deities. There are two different ideas of the relationship between this trio. In both the Very Gracious extends straight up through the torso from the base of the spine to the crown at the thousand-spoke wheel. In one version Comfort and Tawny bow away from Very Gracious, the former at the left side and the latter at the right. In the other version, the two twine around Very Gracious, sometimes compared to the pair of serpents that spiral around what was originally a herald's staff—the caduceus, carried by the Greek god Hermes. Wherever the two nadis cross each other and Very Gracious, we find a cakra. In either case, Tawny ends at the solar right nostril, breathing through which heats the body, while Comfort ends at the lunar left nostril, breathing through which cools the body.

Occasionally, a text will increase the number of major nadis to 12 or 14, the 10 listed already with two or four added on: She Who Flows (*sarasvati*), World Belly (*vishvodara*, also spelled *vishva udara*), Watery (*payasvini*), and *varuna*, which in later mythology became a kind of Indian Neptune or Poseidon, and known as the "lord of sea and rivers."

Though World Belly seems like it belongs among the strange names, it's actually quite appropriate. According to the *Yoga Yajnavalkya*, the "Nadi Vishvodara is situated in the middle of the belly,"[12] or the navel, which places it at the center of the microcosm's world.

I won't try to describe the location of the nadis because different texts arrange them in different ways. In general, though, the main nadis connect to all parts of the body, the eyes and ears, the nose, and the big toes, for example. Of the main nadis, the YY says that they and "various other channels that originate from them are similar to the (pattern of the) veins on the leaf of a pupil (sic) tree or lotus plant."[13]

10 PRANA WINDS (*VAYU*)

The air itself is only the body of another, far more subtle air.

Joseph Joubert (1797)

Just as fish swim in an ocean of water, we swim in an ocean of air that gradually dissipates into airless space. But according to the yogis, there's another ocean in which we swim that permeates everywhere, out to the ends of the universe—if there is one—and this is prana. The word *prana* consists of the prefix *pra-*, "forth" (cognate with the English *fore*), and the verb *ana*, "to breathe." Literally then, *prana* means "to breathe forth," but though breath and prana are closely linked, they're not the same. "Prana is not just breath but is the basic force of life responsible for activating the psycho-physical body, including breath."[14] N. C. Panda describes prana as the "single unitary Being," a "substrate of the empirical multiple entities," in other words, of the material world. Panda summarizes a hymn from the AV dedicated to prana, which tells us the "universe is subject to *Prana* who is the Lord of all and on whom all is supported. He is the Lord of both the living and the non-living creation."[15]

Prana has two levels of existence, the all-pervading *mukhya* (the "principal," or "chief" prana) and the *vyasti* (or individual prana). When we take in air, we also take in prana, at which point it separates into 10 different winds (*vayu*): five major and five minor, each of the former five with its own locus in the body and each of the 10 with its own chore to manage. *Vayu* by the way is rooted in *va*, "to blow," and is cognate with the English word *wind*.

Prana vayu is appropriation, it takes in and inspires, it's centered in the heart, while apana vayu is elimination, expiration, centered in the pelvis. In between these two, centered in the belly, is samana vayu, the "fire in the belly," which stands for assimilation or digestion. It integrates into the body the beneficial substances appropriated by prana vayu and sends the nonessential to apana vayu to be eliminated. Finally udana vayu is centered in the throat as force behind speech, and vyana vayu is diffused throughout the body and controls circulation.

I must admit that I've never quite been able to see the point of the minor vayus (*upaprana*). If we look in a few different texts, we'll find the chores of the minor vayus are inconsistent. Here I'll list them and their various chores. Naga ("serpent") is responsible for belching and vomiting; kurma ("tortoise") is responsible for blinking or closing the eyes; deva datta ("god given") is responsible for sleep or yawning; dhanam jaya ("conquest of wealth") is responsible for hiccuping or swelling the corpse, though the Sanskrit-English dictionary, against all other reference sources, says this prana "nourishes the body." Krikara ("partridge") is the most inconsistently described of the five: it's responsible for either "twinkling of the eyelids," belching, vomiting, hunger and thirst, or sneezing.

SIX WHEELS (*CAKRA*): THE CAKRA SYSTEM

A common mistranslation of cakra is "energy center"; cakras represent particular forms of consciousness and are not merely physical energy centers.

Rajiv Malhotra and Satyanarayana Dasa Babaji, *Sanskrit Non-Translatables: The Importance of Sanskritizing English*

There are certain elements of traditional yoga that have been reworked for a modern audience. Among the most common of these elements are the six cakras. (Sometimes the sahasrara at the crown is included as a cakra, making seven, but sometimes not.) These cakras are usually pictured as ranging along the sushumna nadi, encased in our physical spine, from the sacrum to the lower belly to the navel to the center of the chest (the heart) to the throat to the bridge of the nose. Each is depicted as a lotus flower with a specific number of petals, increasing from four at the base to 16 at the throat. The cakra at the bridge of the nose has only two petals, but the sahasrara at the crown has a thousand.

Each cakra is a powerful symbol, hosting a pair of gods, male and female. Each may be holding some kind of a weapon (e.g., trident, sphere, club) or other item (e.g., conch, waterpot, flower), or forming a hand or two into a mudra (each deity usually has four arms). They're accompanied by a totem animal (e.g., elephant, crocodile, ram), a geometric shape (e.g., square, triangle, quarter moon), each shape with particular color (e.g., the root cakra has a yellow square), and a seed mantra consisting of a Sanskrit consonant meant to be chanted.

As you may be aware, most modern representations of the cakras have stripped away much of this symbolism or changed it in some significant way. Usually all that's shown is the outline of the petaled circle, with a geometric shape and maybe the seed mantra. Gone are the deities, animals, weapons and whatnot, and the colors have been changed to those of the light spectrum or rainbow, red at the base, purple at the crown. In other words, we moderns have simplified the cakras until they no longer come close to resembling their original makeup.

What would a rock-ribbed traditionalist have to say about these changes, not only to the cakras, but to other hallowed elements of the yoga tradition? I can imagine a range of responses: maybe nothing more than a philosophical, what-do-you-expect shrug—times change and yoga must change with them—to a fiery tirade against the distortions and indignities visited on the tradition by Western cultural appropriation.

▸ ▸ BEHIND THE NUMBERS

Other Cakra Systems

Many of us believe that, based on what we've learned from the YS, there are, for example, eight limbs and five yamas and five niyamas in a yoga system. As we'll see in subsequent chapters, this is mistaken: there are yoga systems with fewer and more than eight limbs, and we can find many more yamas and niyamas in the literature.

Similar to this, we also tend to believe that a cakra system has six (or seven) cakras—again a mistake. There are other systems that have more than six or seven cakras. For example, the *Kaula Jnana Nirnaya* (KJN) lists eight cakras[16] and also mentions cakras, visualized as lotuses, with 10,000,000 or 30,000,000 petals. The SSP mentions nine cakras.[17] Akshaya Kumar Banerjea writes that these cakras "represent particular planes of spiritual experience,"[18] that can serve as steps up to the ultimate goal or obstacles to that goal.

◂ ◂

Six in Sanskrit

The Sanskrit word for six is *shash*, though this spelling will change when it's used as a prefix to other words. Without going into the arcane rules of Sanskrit juncture, the two most common spellings of *shash* when used as a prefix are *shat*—as in *shat cakra*, "six wheels"—and *shad*—as in *shad darshana*, "six views."

In the cosmic realm, Vedanta tells us there are six eternals (*anadi*, "having no beginning, existing from eternity"): Brahman (the Absolute), Ishvara (God), the individual Self (*jiva*), Self-ignorance (*avidya*), the difference between *jiva* and *Ishvara*, and the relation between pure consciousness (*cit*) and *avidya* (i.e., consciousness with content).

Existence has six developments (*shad bhava vikara*), which we all have been through, are going through, and will someday inevitably go through: being or existence (*asti*, "is"), birth or coming into being (*jayate*), growth (*vardha*), ripeness or maturity (*parinama*), decline or decay (*kshiyana*), and dissolution or destruction (*nashyat*). Existence also has six waves (*shad urmayah*), of which I found two slightly different versions. But true to some yogis' attitude toward existence, we find no joy or fulfillment in either sets of waves. In both we find hunger (*ashana*) and thirst (*pipasa*), which may be taken literally as a craving for food and drink, but also figuratively as cravings for life. For one version the other four waves are sorrow (*shoka*), delusion (*moha*), dotage (*jara*), and death (*mriti*). For the other version, the four are cold and heat (which apply to the physical body) and greediness and illusion (which apply to the mind).

We have many helpers in our yoga practice, but we have some enemies too—six of them to be exact (*ari shad varga*). Watch out for lust (*kama*), anger (*krodha*), greed (*lobha*), delusion (*moha*), pride (*mada*), and a word that does double duty, *matsarya*, which can mean either "jealousy" (which is what we feel when something we value, often a relationship, is threatened by another person) or "envy" (which is what we feel when something we desire but lack is enjoyed by someone else). We also must contend with six demonic qualities (*asurisampat*): ostentation (*dambha*), arrogance (*darpa*), self-conceit (*abhimana*), anger (*krodha*), harsh language (*parushya*), and spiritual ignorance (*ajnana*).

The *Hatha Yoga Pradipika* provides us with two lists of six, one of don'ts and the other of dos, as its version of *yamas* and *niyamas*. The former includes behaviors that might be called over the top: overeating (*atyahara*); overexertion (*prayasa*); talking too much (*prajalpa*); "seizing vows"—that is, severe austerities (*niyama graha*); "addiction to people" (*jana sanga*), that is, too much socializing; and *laulya*, a word with several possible interpretations: "fickleness, restlessness, greediness, unsteadiness."[19] The dos include enthusiasm or zeal (*utsaha*), boldness or daring (*sahasa*), constancy (*dhairya*), true knowledge (*tattva jnana*), determination (*nishcaya*), and renouncing socializing (*jana sanga paricaya*).

Finally, there are six steps to approach the deity for protection (*shadvidha sharanagati*): to conceive what's in conformity with god's will (*anukulyasya sankalpa*); to reject what's disagreeable (*pratikulyasya varjanam*); to have faith that god will save the Self (*rakshishyatiti vishvasa*); to experience the feeling you're incapable of following the prescribed path of action (*karma*), knowledge (*jnana*), and devotion (*bhakti*) (*karpanya*); to seek god alone as protector (*goptritva varanam*); and to meekly surrender to god (*atma nikshepa*).[20]

◄ ◄

THREE KNOTS (*GRANTHI*)

When the knots are all cut,
that bind our heart to earth;
Then a mortal becomes immortal. . . .
Katha Upanishad 6.15

Granthi is a Sanskrit word for "knot," with the implication that it's not your ordinary knot, but one that is tightly tied and would be challenging to undo. When we read the word *knot*, it's likely the first thing that comes to mind is how we tie the laces of our boots or shoes. But in relation to yoga, the knots are blockages of our subtle energy that restrain or obstruct the free movement of that energy through our subtle body.

The knots have different stories in different texts. The earliest knot stories I found are in three of the 13 (sometimes 14) classical Upanishads, ancient proponents (along with the BG and VS) of monistic Vedanta. The earliest of these early stories is in the *Chandogya Upanishad* (CU), compiled sometime between 800 and 600 BCE. Here Sanatkumara addresses the sage Narada, who calls himself, despite his great learning, a "man full of sorrow," and begs to be taught how to cross to the "other side of sorrow."[21] The answer Sanatkumara gives seems odd, because it doesn't include all the usual suspects—there's no asana, no pranayama, not even meditation. Instead he advises eating pure food, which is supposed to ignite a chain reaction—the food purifies our being, which in turn purifies and strengthens our memory of the Self, and then "all the knots are cut away."[22] I must admit I'm not convinced by this solution, but it does emphasize the importance the yogis place on good nutrition in their practice.

What are these knots, and how do they form? The fifth-century BCE KU explains they're what bind our heart, our essential Self, securely to the mundane world and our illusory ideas of who we are.[23] The knots are inevitable accompaniments of our own Self-ignorance, that result in bondage to our limited self, and they must be cut if we're ever to reclaim our true Self.

A third Upanishad, the third- or second-century BCE *Mundaka Upanishad*, proposes a second way to cut the knots: simply reveal our true Self, right now sequestered in the "cave of the heart," the innermost sanctum of our being.[24] With this cutting, continues MuU, all doubts about the Self are "dispelled" and it "becomes visible as the immortal / in the form of bliss."[25] This solution seems to me as questionable as the first. It makes revealing the Self sound like a walk in the park, but we know it's far more challenging than that.

Upon the appearance of Hindu Tantra around 500 to 600 CE and continuing with its offspring Hatha Yoga arriving maybe 300 years later, the indeterminate number of knots in the Upanishads become three (*tri granthi*). They're each settled in a new home, in one of three of the six purported energy wheels (*cakra*) distributed along the spine of our subtle body. From its origin in the bulb (*kanda*) near the perineum, sushumna rises through its physical counterpart to the atlas, the first cervical vertebra, then beyond to terminate at the crown.

The three wheels that concern us are the first, fourth, and fifth (though some texts situate the first knot in the third cakra). Their names are Muladhara ("root-support," at the level of the sacrum), Anahata ("unstruck," at the level of the sternum), and Vishuddha ("pure," at the level of the throat). Once installed in their new abodes, knots will be knots, and so all three go right back to knotting things up just as their predecessors did in the heart.

It's beyond the scope of this text to describe in detail the cakras and the process and ultimate goal of the Tantra-Hatha project. Just briefly then, the subtle body is our unseen inner world, crisscrossed by a highly complex network of tens of thousands of energy channels (*nadi*). At the center of this network, like the hub of a wheel, is the sushumna, the most important of all the channels, with its six cakras. (Again, the wheel at the crown is also sometimes identified as a cakra, making seven total.)

The heroine of this world is represented by a coiled serpent, reminiscent of a compressed spring, a symbol of unlimited potential energy waiting to be unleashed. Asleep at the base of the spine, her mouth covers (and so blocks) the entrance to sushumna, the only one of the myriad channels whose entry is barred. Ironically, it's precisely the one channel we want to have open, since it gives the serpent access to the path she's meant to follow to the crown for our Self-realization. The serpent is us— or it might be more exact to say she's our spiritual potential, her slumber our Self-ignorance. Like the knots, the serpent is an ambiguous symbol, both the cause of our worldly bondage and, when awakened, our ride through sushumna to the top where freedom awaits.

And there's the rub. By all accounts, waking the serpent and driving it along sushumna's channel is hard enough, but throw in the knots as additional obstacles and we have before us a journey fraught with dangers, our success by no means assured. Many texts warn us in no uncertain terms not to make this journey solo, but first to secure the assistance of an experienced guide in the form of a guru.

The knots are named after the deities in the Hindu trimurti: the Brahma knot binds the first cakra, Vishnu the fourth, and Rudra (an early appellation of Shiva) the fifth. In this story, it's at these knots, writes John Woodroffe in his classic study of kundalini, *The Serpent Power*, that the "force of Maya Shakti is in great strength"[26] What's Maya Shakti? Woodroffe explains that she's "that which seemingly makes the Whole . . . into the not-whole, the infinite into the finite, the formless into forms and the like." She's the power that "cuts down, veils, and negates"[27] our perfect consciousness, which alienates us from our true Self—in a word, avidya (see chapter 2).

There are other versions of the knot story in texts dedicated either to Shiva or Shakti. We'll have to pass on these for the time being. More research is needed to complete this project.

The Hatha knot-cutting techniques are no more satisfying to me than the two from the Upanishads. They're either too esoteric or too aggressive. I did, however, come across an approach propounded by Lama Anagarika Govinda that seems both reasonable and effective. My only hesitation is that it comes from a Tibetan Buddhism perspective and is applied in a slightly different context—there are, for example, six knots. I've nothing against Tibet or Buddhism; what worries me is that a practice shouldn't for the most part be used out of its context. Still, I think it's worth our consideration, not only for cutting knots but for welcoming life as well. It's also a beautifully written story, so I quote it at length.

The lama says we must reverse the "coagulation of consciousness into a state of materiality"[28] by untying the knots one by one from Muladhara upward to the crown.

It is therefore not a question of gaining or creating miraculous powers, but only of restoring the disturbed equilibrium of our psychic forces, by freeing ourselves from our inner tensions and our mental and spiritual crampedness. This can only be achieved through a relaxed, serene, and blissful state of body and soul, but not through self-mortification, asceticism . . . , or through violation of body and mind by way of artificial breathing exercises and strenuous efforts to fetter the mind to preconceived ideas.[29]

Tradition tells us when the knots are cut we can expect to hear certain sounds for each one in the right ear. Cutting the Brahma knot produces the "sweet tinkling sound of ornaments . . . in the ethereal void . . . of the heart." Cutting the Vishnu produces sounds "like those of a kettle-drum," and cutting the Rudra will also produce a "drum-like sound."[30]

Going through all that trouble to cut the knots and being rewarded with drumming in your right ear seems rather anticlimactic. Ajit Mookerjee has a modern and far more satisfying view on what to expect. When the Brahma is cut, we "get established in totality"; when the Vishnu is cut, we'll see the "existence of a universal life-principle"; and finally when the Rudra is cut we'll "attain the non-dual state, realization of oneness, the universal joy."[31]

TRIPLE BRAID (*TRIVENI*)

Here (within this body) is the Ganges and the Jumna. . . . Here are Prayaga and Banaras. . . . Here are the sacred places. . . . I have not seen a place of pilgrimage and an abode of bliss like my body.

Saraha, *Dohakosha*

Allahabad is a city in northern India, also known historically as Prayaga, the "place of sacrifice." It's at the confluence (*samgama*) of two great rivers, the Ganges and Yamuna, or three if you count the Sarasvati, "she who flows"—a river no one's actually ever seen. Out of respect, let's just say she's fabled, made more so because her bed is said to be underground and she somehow joins the other two from below. To purify their souls, many pilgrims come here to bathe in what's called the triple braid (*triveni*), that holiest confluence of three rivers, the white Ganges, the blue Yamuna, and the mysterious, subterranean, invisible Sarasvati.

▸ ▸ STORY

"She Who Flows": Sarasvati, the Mythical River

Controversy swirls around the Sarasvati. Four thousand years ago, she may have run down from the Himalayas southward across what's now the Thar Desert in western India, emptying into the Gulf of Kutch and the Arabian Sea. The RV tells us that in her day, she surpassed in "majesty and might all other waters,"[32] and was possibly the lifeline of a thriving civilization.

It's speculated that sometime before 1900 BCE, something catastrophic happened—maybe a widespread tectonic upheaval that changed its course or the end of the yearly monsoons that fed it brought on by climate change—and the Sarasvati slowed to a trickle and dried up. Her exact course, the manner of her demise, and even if she ever existed are matters of some debate. There's also the bothersome question of how she managed to migrate over 800 miles eastward to meet up with her two companions at Prayaga.

There have also been many attempts to identify the former riverbed. Scientists studying this question believe the Sarasvati ran through the Thar Desert in western India, but others believe this was a myth from the very beginning. However she dried up, whether she was or wasn't, and however she turned east, today the Sarasvati exists only in the collective imagination of the Indian people.

◂ ◂

Whatever the true story is, the triveni made by the three rivers is acclaimed throughout India, and the braid has been the chosen destination of pilgrims and seekers for a very long time. That's because the triveni is also a *tirtha*. Literally, a tirtha is either a "passage" or "ford," a shallow river crossing where travelers can wade safely to the other side or a bathing-place. But in India, such sites are often reframed spiritually. The BG, for example, takes place on the eve of the apocalyptic battle on "field of the Kurus," the Kurukshetra. This battlefield was in time homologized with the human body, where in each of us the struggle rages, of which we are mostly unaware, between the forces of ignorance and insight to block or realize the Self. Similarly, the tirtha was recast as a sacred bridge linking two worlds, the mundane with the divine.

Each of us, as a miniature recreation of the universe, has a triveni and several tirthas. The former, not coincidentally, is situated at the bridge of the nose where our three main subtle energy channels twine together for the last time. The ida nadi is equated with the Ganges, the pingala with the Yamuna, and interestingly enough, the Sarasvati with the central sushumna nadi.

Just as India spiritualizes the world, it also tends to internalize external rituals, even to the point of criticizing their external performance. The "true meaning of the ritual is not to be found in outer action . . . [but] realized within the self, through the knowledge of the ritual's inner meaning and the withdrawal of the senses from the sensory world."[33] So we have the *Darshana Upanishad* (DU) telling us that if we abandon our internal tirthas for the external ones, it's like going "after pieces of glass abandoning the precious gems" we hold in our hands.

> Do not resort to Tirthas filled with water, nor gods made of wood and the like . . . the internal Tirtha is the Tirtha by far superior to external Tirtha.[34]

According to the DU, we have tirthas at our crown, forehead, bridge of the nose (but not in this text); the *triveni*, which is located in the subtle heart center (*anahata cakra*) in close proximity to two other tirthas; and lastly in the sacrum.

▸ ▸ PRACTICE

Triple Braid and the Interior Pilgrimage

The bridge of the nose is also the traditional site of several other subtle structures or organs. There we might find the clairvoyant divine eye (*divya cakshus*) or the wisdom eye (*jnana cakshus*), which can, unlike the physical eye, perceive the Self.[35] There too is the sixth cakra, the "wheel of command" (*ajna cakra*), beautifully bright "like the Moon."[36] If we meditate on this center, we can realize our "unity with Brahman," and become the "benefactor of all."[37]

The anonymous author of the DU invites us to go on a pilgrimage to tirthas inside our own body. Pilgrimage was an essential ingredient of traditional Indian life. It was undertaken for a variety of reasons, often though to atone for sin or to erase some accumulated karma. Undertaking a pilgrimage in our own body is considerably more convenient than traveling to India, and apparently, in the DU author's opinion, considerably more effective than pilgrimages to external tirthas.

He suggests seven destinations as focal points for our meditations: Shri Parvata, the name of a mountain, appropriately located at the crown; Kedara, the name of a mountainous area in the Himalayas, in our forehead; the holy city of Benares at the bridge of the nose; in the chest is the "field of the Kurus," Kurukshetra, a large plain near Delhi and the setting of the BG and the great battle that followed; our own personal Prayaga in the lotus of the heart (*anahata cakra*); Cidambaram (the "ether of consciousness") in the middle of the heart; Kamalalaya (the "abode of the lotuses") in the Muladhara (the "root-support," the base cakra).

The anonymous author of the *Yoga Shikha Upanishad* (YSU) has a different destination in mind for the interior pilgrimage: the single most important nadi. Just as Shiva's 8,400,000 asanas were pared down to one (see p. 137), likewise the 72,000 nadis are reduced to the Most Gracious channel, sushumna nadi, to which he urges us make our pilgrimage.

The Sushumna alone is the holiest place of pilgrimage. . . . The Sushumna alone is meditation of the highest order. The Sushumna alone is the worthiest goal. The various kinds of sacrifices, gifts, vows and austere observances do not deserve even a sixteenth part of the merit due to Yoga attained by meditating on the Sushumna.[38]

You might sit or recline, close your eyes, and bring all of your attention to the tirtha at the bridge of your nose. Bathing in a tirtha is said to be a transformative occasion, so you might visualize the three nadis as the confluence of the three rivers, and imaginatively wade into it up to waist height. Traditional bathing is a rather solemn procedure, accompanied with sacred materials, ritual gestures, and mantras, and since I assume most readers of this book aren't Hindus, I believe it would be inappropriate to mimic what's done. For this exercise then, simply remain as conscious as possible as you mentally scoop up the water of these rivers in your cupped hands and rub it gently over your torso.

◄ ◄

6

HATHA YOGA
BY THE NUMBERS

The term *hatha* is from the root *hath* meaning "to treat with violence" or "to oppress," and hence, the expression "Hatha Yoga" means something like "the discipline of bodily exertion."
Gerald James Larson and Ram Shankar Bhattacharya,
Encyclopedia of Indian Philosophies, vol. 12, *Yoga:
India's Philosophy of Meditation,* "Introduction"

Among the many little oddities about traditional texts, one that always amuses me is their penchant for predicting the time it will take the practitioner to arrive at his desired destination, whether it's the mastering of an individual practice or of Self-ignorance (*avidya*). We have an example of this in the *Shiva Samhita* (SS) informing the mridu student that they can expect a 12-year journey to their goal. In none of these estimated times of arrival at perfection (ETAPs) is there any consideration of the traveler themself, their abilities or intensity of practice. I suppose, just to be kind to the mostly anonymous authors, we can say they were trying to keep their practitioners' expectations within reasonable bounds and that the numbers they presented were perhaps averages: some high-powered mridus could possibly succeed within eight years; the more casual ones—if it's even possible for a mridu to be any more casual—16 years.

The next rung up is the middling (*madhya*) practitioner. In every way, he is ... well, "average," "normal," "levelheaded"—and here's where I take offense—"like those who have reached middle age."[1] Reading about him is soporific. He's directed to Laya Yoga, the yoga of dissolution, and can expect to muddle his way to perfection in eight years.

After the rather unimpressive lead-off pair—the latter one excused, of course, because of being middle-aged—we come to the "above measure" (*adhimatra*) practitioner. This one seems more like the traditional yogi we're accustomed to: steady-minded, energetic, magnanimous, sympathetic, truthful, courageous. There's lots more, but I think you get the picture. Their practice is Hatha Yoga, and they will need half the time of the mridu—that is, six years—to succeed.

Lastly, we have the superstar among the four: this one is also adhimatra, but with the suffix *-tama* attached (*adhimatratama*), which makes the student superlative. If we thought the previous practitioner seemed very close to perfection, the superlative practitioner seems to have crossed the perfection line—at least from my perspective down near the bottom of the ladder, though I am past middle age. Reading about the *-tama* suffixed *adhimatra*—heroic, clean, skillful, competent, talented, peaceful, and naturally "in the prime" of their youth—we have to wonder why they even need a yoga practice at all. At this level, they are entitled to take their pick of any yoga school they prefer, and their ETAP is three years. But we have to wonder too why it will take them so long to reach their goal.

▸ ▸ STORY

The Origin of Hatha Yoga

Once upon a time there was a fisherman who, out in his boat on the sea one day, was pulled overboard and swallowed by a huge fish—usually described as a whale, though of course a whale isn't a fish. Stuck inside the fish's belly, the fisherman was transported to isolated Moon Island.

Coincidentally at that time Shiva and Shakti were also there on the island so the former could instruct the latter in the secrets of yoga far away from prying ears. But they didn't get far enough away, at least if you've taken up residence in a fish's belly. While Shakti fell asleep during her husband's peroration, the fisherman took it all in. Shiva, suspecting that Shakti wasn't paying the closest attention, asked her: "Are you listening?" and the fisherman, who was listening very carefully, replied without thinking, "Yes!" Shiva, realizing he'd been overheard and pleased with the fisherman's rapt attention, initiated him as Matsyendra, the "Lord of the Fish," into the secrets of his teaching.

Matsyendra then either emerged immediately from the fish's belly or decided to stay put and, after 12 years of refining his practice, was freed by a fellow fisherman who had trapped the great marine animal and cut open its belly. Matsyendra then became the first human teacher of Hatha Yoga.

◂ ◂

FOUR LEVELS OF ASPIRANTS

Know that aspirants are of four orders:—mild (*mridu*), moderate (*madhya*), ardent (*adhimatra*), and supremely ardent (*adhimatratama*)—the best who can cross the ocean of existence.

Shiva Samhita 5.13

Traditional Hatha Yoga delineates four levels of students in ascending order, each with a practice appropriate to the level. At the bottom of the ladder is the *mridu* student; the kindest way to translate the Sanskrit is "mild." The SS—which frankly tends to be a bit rigid in some of its attitudes—draws a rather unappealing portrait of mridu.[2] Let's just say this student is sorely lacking in many areas deemed important by the anonymous author, who isn't inclined to cut mridu any slack. He's directed to practice Mantra Yoga and can expect to succeed "with great efforts" after 12 years.

▸ ▸ BEHIND THE NUMBERS

Two Meanings of Hatha

Probably the most widely known figurative definition comes from the YSU. Many experienced students, if questioned about Hatha's meaning, will respond with "Sun Moon," though they're not always perfectly clear about what this refers to.

To arrive at this definition, *Hatha* is divided into its two syllables, *ha* and *tha*, the former assigned the meaning of "sun," the latter "moon." These are the two great lights in our sky, and like everything in the macrocosm, they have equivalents in the microcosm of our body (see chapter 2). The sun correlates to our heating energy; the moon is cooling. In Patanjali's world they're a "pair of opposites" (*dvandva*),[3] along with many others like wet-dry, light-dark, up-down. These pairs are forever pulling us to and fro as if we were the rope in a game of tug-of-war. This contributes to those unwanted fluctuations of consciousness (*citta vrittis*) that obscure the Self, often compared to the way roiling the water of an otherwise placid, clear pool blocks a view of the pool's bottom. One of the characteristics of a successfully performed asana is the quieting of this pair and any others that disturb our peace of mind.

Hatha Yoga has a much different take on the sun and moon. This school equates the pair with the two nadis that spiral around the central subtle energy channel of the sushumna nadi. The sun is the heating, Tawny pingala nadi that terminates in the right nostril; the moon the cooling, Comfort ida nadi that terminates in the left. Rather than withdraw from them, which is the long-term strategy of Patanjali in regard to the physical world, the Hatha yogi wants to integrate the two, to join their energies together to create a union.

Now if we compare "Sun Moon" to the dictionary definition at the head of the chapter, we get a hint of how this union in Hatha Yoga is achieved. *Hatha* is literally "force, violence" (as well as "obstinacy, pertinacity"), which may be interpreted in two ways: Hatha Yoga can be translated as Forceful Yoga, or alternatively, Yoga of the Force (i.e., Kundalini) or Kundalini Yoga. When I have occasion to mention this literal meaning to a roomful of students, there are often at least a few who express surprise. All along they've believed that Hatha is defined by its figurative etymology.

◄ ◄

Two Meanings of Guru

> The syllable *Gu* indicates darkness, the syllable *Ru* means its dis-
> peller. Because of the quality of dispelling darkness, the Guru is
> so termed.
>
> *Advaya Taraka Upanishad* 16

The word *guru*, like *hatha*, has both a figurative and a literal definition.
As we can see in the *Advaya Taraka Upanishad* (ATU), the two syllables
of the word are interpreted as darkness (*gu*) and light (*ru*), so it's said
that the guru guides us from the darkness of Self-ignorance to the light
of Self-knowing.[4] It's also written about the two syllables that the guru
is totally free because he's beyond both the three qualities (*gunas*, see p.
36) of nature (*gu*) and all of its forms (*ru*, which suggests *rupa*, form).[5]
Finally, the guru possesses the supreme knowledge (*ru*) that destroys all
illusion (*gu*).[6]

The syllable *gu* is also related to *go*, the Sanskrit word for "cow."
The guru thus feeds the student like the cow her calf. This association
also suggests the great "spotted cow," a symbol of the divine store of life
energy: "Through the continuous transformation into the energy and
substance of the world the infinite store suffers not the least decrease.
The cow suffers no diminution, either of life-substance or of productive
vigor."[7]

The word's literal meaning is much different. *Guru* is "heavy,
weighty," the image of one loaded down with spiritual wisdom. *Guru* is
also "important, serious, momentous; valuable, highly prized; any ven-
erable or respectable person (father, mother, or any relative older than
oneself); a spiritual parent or preceptor (from whom a youth receives
the initiatory mantra or prayer)." As we can see, a guru isn't to be trifled
with.

◂ ◂

TYPES OF GURU

The Guru is Brahman, the Guru is Vishnu; the Guru is always the Lord Acyuta; greater than the Guru there is no one whatsoever in all the three worlds. One should worship with extreme devotion (the Guru), who imparts divine wisdom, who is the spiritual guide, who is the Supreme Lord (himself).

Yoga Shikha Upanishad 5.56–57

If you wanted a yoga education in traditional India, you needed a guru. "Although many of the yoga traditions have textual foundations, the real foundation of the teaching of yoga is the guru. The practice of yoga is not traditionally learned from books, but from personal instruction."[8]

As you can see in the epigraph—and we can find many more like it in the literature—the guru wasn't considered to be an average person. Nowadays in the West, the word *guru* is used rather loosely to designate a mentor or an expert in a particular field or endeavor. We also see it in names for everything from bicycles to energy drinks to apps for buying a previously owned car or securing an aisle seat on an airplane. But in ancient India the title wasn't handed out willy-nilly; instead, it was strictly reserved for a special type of spiritual teacher revered as a god incarnate.

You might have noticed that I didn't put a specific number down for the types of guru in the heading for this section. We might think a guru is a guru is a guru, but that's not the case. Just as yoga has different schools, these schools recognize different types of gurus. The number three is common, which might be seen as a reflection of the trimurti (see p. 51) as hinted at in the epigraph—though Shiva, oddly enough, isn't included (*acyuta*, "never falling," is a nickname for Vishnu). A trio from the BVU is identified as the prompter or "impeller" (*codaka*), who points the way to liberation through meditation; the awakener (*bodhaka*), who rouses the strong belief in the student of their identity with Brahman; and finally the "giver" of liberation (*moksha*), the "transcendent Brahman" itself, which imparts to the student the truth, "All is of my form. . . . There is not even a speck beyond me."[9] Knowing this, according to the BVU, "one attains immortality." The Upanishad nonetheless doesn't make it clear how an unliberated individual is able to contact Brahman and enlist its help.

Just for contrast, the *Kularnava Tantra* (KT) names six gurus, without giving much detail about their roles. They are the *preraka* ("setting in motion, urging"), who apparently gets the ball rolling; the *sucaka*, an interesting word meaning both "pointing out, teacher," and "treacherous, villain," presumably the first rendering applies here; *vacaka*, "speaker"; *darshaka*, "showing, pointing out"; *sikshaka*, "teaching, one who knows"; and *bodhaka*, "awakening."[10]

‣ ‣ BEHIND THE NUMBERS

Do We Really Need a Guru to Practice Yoga Successfully?

As a sidenote, it may have once been universally agreed that an aspirant couldn't succeed without a guru, and even today there are people who feel the same. But not everybody does. One of the most notable nay-sayers was the late Indian sage Jiddu Krishnamurti: "Another can point out the way, but you have to do all the work, even if you have a guru. . . . No one can lead you to the truth; and if anyone leads you, it can only be to the known."[11] In Krishnamurti's world, the "known" is another word for bondage, so his meaning is clear: to find the truth, a guru's help is limited—it can only take us to the boundary of the known. In the end, to pass that boundary is a step we have to take by ourselves. We'll skip over the question of whether or not Krishnamurti was himself a guru, though he insisted he wasn't.

◂ ◂

What qualities might we look for when deciding whether or not this or that person makes the grade as a true guru? The KT spins out a whole laundry list of a guru's desirable characteristics,[12] and suffice it to say that someone who embodies even half is a remarkable human being. I think that one verse here sums it all up: "He who makes us know: 'I am the knower of the essence of all teachings, I am the core, who is inseparable (from *Brahman*) and who is ever-pleased in heart'—he [who does that] is the Guru."[13]

Another text, the *Laws of Manu*, informs us in great detail what we should and shouldn't do in and out of the guru's presence. It's clear the student is expected to treat his godlike guru with the kind of kow-towing reverence reserved in our time for rock and movie stars, super-wealthy business moguls, and cult leaders. Punishments for dissing the guru were severe to say the least, even extending beyond one's current incarnation. Speak ill of your guru, warns Manu, and in your next life you'll be reborn as a donkey. You'll wind up with a dog's life, literally, if you reproach the guru (and Fido wasn't the pampered pooch we find in most families today; he was considered "unclean" and treated poorly), a worm's life if you mooch off him, and an unspecified bug's life if you begrudge him.[14]

Even so, it was understood, as it still is today, that not all gurus are exemplars of fine behavior. We're advised to abandon gurus who delude us by means of their scriptural knowledge, who are ignorant, who don't tell the truth or are hypocritical.[15] Certainly we can add to this short list that we should immediately reject a guru—or any teacher for that matter—who makes unreasonable financial demands or who is verbally or physically abusive.

TYPES OF INITIATION (*DIKSHA*)

It is through initiation that . . . man becomes what he is and what he should be—a being open to the life of the spirit.

Mircea Eliade, *Myths, Rites, Symbols*

Every four years, in Olympia, Greece, the Olympic flame is lighted a few months before the start of the competition. When the time comes, it's transported, by a circuitous route, to the site of that year's games, usually—but not always—by a relay of runners.

This is much like the story of how the traditional teachings of Hatha Yoga were passed along from one generation to the next. Most yoga schools trace their beginning to mythic age and a divine source, when the lineage's first teacher, the *adiguru*, received the imprimatur of the lineage's favored deity. For Hatha Yoga, the original flame is the *adinatha*, the "primal lord"—Shiva, the patron saint of Hatha. By tradition, Shiva passed the teachings on to Matsyendra, and when his leg of the journey was done, Matsyendra did the same to his successor, and so on down the line. There's a list of these runners—32 in all—at HYP 1.5–9. It's called a *parampara*, "proceeding from one to another"—in a word, a lineage. Here though, the teachings have no destination, and instead, they'll be handed off endlessly from runner to runner to the end of time.

The basic concept of initiation and the word *diksha* date back to the AV, at least 3,000 years ago. The initiation is compared to a birth: the "Master," as the symbolic mother, welcomes his "new disciple," the symbolic child, "into his bowels," and for three nights "he holds and bears him in this belly. When he is born, the Gods convene to see him,"[16] which no doubt makes for a momentous occasion.

Initiation was an indispensable event in a yogi's life. Historian of religion Mircea Eliade writes that it "represents one of the most significant spiritual phenomena in the history of humanity."[17]

Through initiation, the disciple was symbolically reborn into a new mode of being; everything that went before that moment belonged to another life that no longer existed. The guru would now be their only family—mother, father, siblings rolled into one—but more than that, the guru would also be their god incarnate. Every subsequent initiation across the ages was a reenactment of the primal scene, the teacher standing in for the deity, the disciple humbly playing the role of the lineage founder. In this way, the teaching with all its god-infused wisdom and potency is passed along from teacher to student without end. A teacher offering "unsanctified" teaching would land "for many years in the horrible hell," a decidedly unappealing prospect.[18]

It appears that convincing a proper, godly teacher to accept you as a student wasn't that easy. The KT has a list of unacceptable behaviors, character traits, and physical attributes that runs on for 20 verses.[19] Some reasons for rejection are perfectly understandable: people who are treacherous, mean, addicted to gambling, inveterate liars, greedy, who lack compassion and faith need not apply. From our perspective though, it's hard to read that instruction was also denied to people with physical disabilities, who might be vision or hearing impaired or considered ugly.

It's common for traditional texts to begin with a shout-out to the teaching's source. "Salutations to *adinatha*" is how Svatmarama, compiler of the HYP, introduces his work.[20] He recognizes and pays respect to "the lord (*natha*) of beginnings (*adi*)," that is, Shiva. Alternatively, the salute may be directed to a god who can lend a helping hand. Sundara Deva, author of the *Hatha Tatva Kaumudi* (HTK), and Shrinivasa Yogi, author of the *Hatha Ratna Avali* (HRA), both call on Shiva's elephant-headed son Ganesha, the remover of obstacles routinely invoked at the commencement of texts.[21]

Why was it so difficult to get initiated? Zimmer writes that "wisdom, in the Orient, no matter what its kind, is to be guarded jealously and communicated sparingly, and then only to one capable of becoming its perfect receptacle, for besides representing a certain skill, every department of learning carries with it a power that can amount almost to magic, a power to bring to pass what without it would seem a miracle."[22] Such power in the hands of someone unfit to wield it properly would be disastrous. Teachers had to be especially cautious not to accept and instruct ruthless and morally unprincipled people who could unleash these powers to gain their own selfish ends or to cause great harm to others—think Anakin Skywalker.

The student, once initiated, had to swear to keep the teaching "strictly secret."[23] Secrecy set the initiate apart from the uninitiated and enhanced the potency of the practice. Reveal the secret to the uninitiated, and the practice was rendered impotent.

The teachings—it's important to understand—aren't passed along to just anyone. A teaching is only relayed to qualified individuals. Without this initiation, there's no lineage, and without that, there's no way to connect to the source, the original flame. And without that, there's no yoga, at least no traditional yoga.

There are many different kinds and levels of initiation, from the "formal acceptance by the master with minimal rites to more elaborate ritual procedures."[24] Just as the yogis use different modalities for practice—sound, breath, physical posture, and movement—so also do they use different modalities for initiation. For example, the guru might invest their hands with spiritual power drawn from meditating on the deity and then touch the disciple, imbuing them with transformative energy. The guru might install the 48—or 50—letters and syllables of the nagari alpha-syllabary into different limbs and areas of the disciple's body, then withdraw, then reinstall, and the "state of Godhood full of delight is born in the child (of the guru)."[25] This is "likened to the slow nourishing of its young by the bird with the warmth of its wings."[26] There are initiations, among many others, that use mantras or sight, in which the guru closes both eyes, meditates on the "Supreme Truth with a happy mind," then gazes "well into the disciple."[27]

FOUR STAGES (*AVASTHA*) OF YOGA

There are four stages in all Yogas: beginning (*arambha*), pot (*ghata*), accumulation (*paricaya*), and consummation (*nishpatti*).
Hatha Yoga Pradipika 4.69

One goal of most schools of yoga is summed up in one of the meanings of the word *yoga* itself: "union." This word is usually defined as an "act . . . of joining two or more things into one." The two things, or existents in this case, are the embodied Self (*jivatman*) and the supreme Self (*paramatman*). But what appears to us, in our Self-ignorance (*avidya*), as two separate things, in fact have always been and always will be one and the same. It's impossible then for yoga to *create* a union; rather, what yoga does is lower the veil of Self-ignorance that hides the fullness of our true identity to *reveal* the union that's always existed.

Now whenever anyone—yogi or not—has a goal in life, they have two questions: Is what I'm doing to reach my goal effective? And if it is, then how close am I to reaching it? In the mid-fifteenth century, Svatmarama, compiler of the HYP, offered to help answer these questions by proposing a set of four graduated stages he named Beginning (*arambha*), Connection (*ghati*), Accumulation (*paricaya*), and Consummation (*nishpatti*). Svatmarama summarized what a yogi should expect to experience in each of these stages, so they could determine, first of all, if their practice was sufficient to bring them to and then elevate them beyond arambha and, if it was, then second, just where they stood among the remaining three stages.

Svatmarama didn't specifically name the driving force behind the yogi's ascent through the stages. But since it's coordinated with the rise of pranic energy through the central subtle channel or sushumna nadi, one possibility is that the generator is some form of pranayama. As the prana rises, it pierces the knots (*granthi*) located at the heart, throat, and midbrow cakras (see p. 72) and comes to a terminus at the crown, at what's called the "sacred seat" (*sharva pitha*).

A second possibility might be Nada Yoga, the yoga of subtle sound. The eight verses on the stages are embedded in 28 verses on nada, four preceding[28] and 24 following it.[29] Like the rising prana, there's also a clear connection between nada and the stages. Each time a knot is pierced, a subtle sound is heard—if we can even say a subtle sound can be heard, the yogi has to listen extremely carefully—in a void (*shunya*) associated with the knot's cakra. A fourth sound is heard when the prana touches the crown. These sounds are apparently signals, telling the yogi that a certain stage had been reached. They are tinkling in arambha, drumming in both ghata and paricaya, and the plucking of a lute string in nishpatti.

As the yogi ascends through the stages, their body-mind undergoes a radical transformation. In arambha the body and its fragrance are both described as *divya*, which means "beautiful, charming, divine, splendorous." The yogi also becomes disease-free, their heart swells with contentment, and their mind empties and becomes quiet. When the Brahma knot in the heart cakra is pierced, the yogi experiences a "superior blissful feeling" in the void of the heart. So far, so good.

Advancing to the second stage, the yogi's posture (*asana*) becomes firm and resolute (*drdha*), and the prana reaches the *atishunya*, the "extraordinary void" in the throat. Here, where the Vishnu knot is pierced, the yogi's wisdom expands beyond human bounds. They then also hear a drumming sound, which heralds the supreme bliss to come in paricaya. Now the yogi is *deva samastha*, "equal to the gods." Since the yogi is only at stage 2, this is surprising. Their rise through the ranks from human to the threshold of divinity seems unusually rapid, and we might wonder: What's next? Where can they possibly go from here?

In the third stage, prana passes into the *mahashunya*, the "great void," in the midbrow and pierces the last knot, Rudra. This brings in its wake the supreme bliss (*sahajananda*) promised by the drumming sound in ghata. The yogi now acquires special powers (*siddhi*) and is no longer at the mercy of human frailties; suffering, old age, hunger, and sleep are things of the past. At the same time though, the yogi will now miss out on the pleasures of being human, the intense feeling of relief at the end of a period of suffering, the joys of eating when hungry and sleeping when weary. Old age? That I'm not so sure about.

Finally in nishpatti, when prana reaches the crown, the yogi's consciousness is totally integrated in a state called raja yoga, which besides naming Patanjali's yoga, is also here a synonym for samadhi. Our question in ghata about what's next for an already godlike yogi is answered, and once again a significant promotion is awarded: at the consummation of their ascent the yogi is granted the "power of creating and destroying the whole universe like God himself."[30] This is either enormously impressive or beyond terrifying if true, though we wouldn't be blamed if we were skeptical about this claim.

There are several other versions of Svatmarama's stages spread out over the 300 years or so following the HYP. In that time the practice of yoga inevitably changed, and so did then the expectations for each of the stages, though the names stayed the same. Different methods were used to achieve arambha, such as chanting OM in solitude, the withdrawal of consciousness from the world outside, that is, pratyahara (see p. 148), and a three-month regimen of alternate nostril breathing (*nadi shodhana*), 20 rounds, four times a day at the junctions.

Purification of the Energy Channels (Nadi Shodhana), *Imaginary Version*

Nadi shodhana is usually considered to be a preparation for a formal pranayama practice. There's a very simple way to approximate the practice that can be done either sitting up or lying on a blanket support under your spine.

Sit or lie down and close your eyes. Take a minute or two to observe yourself without judgment or expectation. Then bring your breath into the foreground of your awareness and observe again for a minute or two. Then focus on your left nostril, and imagining the right one blocked, inhale a comfortable amount. Then imagine blocking the left nostril and opening the right, and exhale slowly. Pause and wait for the breath to come back to you.

Then keeping the nostrils as they are, inhale slowly through the right, pause, close the right, open the left and exhale. This completes one round. Continue for a number of rounds or time of your choice. Finish with an exhale through the left nostril and return to everyday breathing, observing your breath again for a minute or two.

◂ ◂

Once within arambha, many of the texts favored pranayama to take the yogi the rest of the way. In nishpatti the consummations differed, though the kind of frightening power granted Svatmarama's yogi was nowhere in sight. But there was plenty of mukti to go around mixed in with some immortality.

What are we to make of all this? Obviously our world and the yogi's are very different places, as are the practices we each favor. As a consequence, the traditional stages aren't much use to us, except historically as backward looks into the early centuries of Hatha Yoga. They do nevertheless teach us three important lessons. First, yoga is always changing, and it's up to us to make sure it always does so for the better. Second, as our practice progresses, our body-mind should get healthier, and anything we do, or are asked to do, in the name of yoga that's unhealthy isn't really yoga. Finally, the ultimate outcome is conditioned by the practice, and since everyone's practice is technically a little bit different, none of us can know exactly how it will all turn out.

7

PRELIMINARY PRACTICES
BY THE NUMBERS

Giving up the seer, seeing and what is seen, along with their impressions (on the mind), seek shelter in the Atman, the first that is manifest in the seeing.

Varaha Upanishad, ii Mantra 18–20

We have at least four different versions of a seven-stage practice that promises to help us move toward Self-realization. With the current version, there's a kind of preliminary stage in which we take a long, searching look at ourselves. Peering "through a glass, darkly," we sense there's something essential missing from our lives, but we can't exactly put our finger on it. We know it's not the usual things we yearn for—I won't even bother to give examples, you know better than I what they are—but we do know for a certainty we'll never be truly happy until we figure out what it is.

To enter the first stage then, we have to admit to and accept our Self-ignorance. We're advised then to begin our practice with the study of sacred texts and to spend time with people who have Self-realized and are willing to help us do the same. The work we do in this pre-stage readies us for the first stage—*shubha iccha*, the "wish" or "desire" (*iccha*) for the "splendid, agreeable, capable, auspicious, virtuous, distinguished, blissful" (*shubha*). At this stage, we're enjoined to perform anonymous deeds of charity and speak wisely, with due respect and love.

Achieving the second stage, we cultivate *vicarana*, "reflection, investigation, inquiry" into the Self. We learn to discriminate between the real and unreal, and like a snake sloughing its outgrown skin, free ourselves of pride, envy, egoism, desires, and delusions. As we distance ourselves from the lure of worldly objects, our consciousness becomes *tanu manasi*, "attenuated" or finely honed to a sharp meditation point. This leads us to the fourth stage of *sattva apatti*, literally "entering into a state (*apatti*) of Truth (*sattva*)" with a capital *T*.

In the fifth stage—*asamsakti*, literally "unconnected"—we simultaneously achieve total nonattachment and insight into the nature of Truth, rejoice in our own Self, and overcome all duality, inside and out. We might note here that the name Svatmarama, the author of the HYP, means "he who delights (*rama*) in his own Self (*sva*)." In the sixth stage or *padartha bhavana*, we realize the essence of life as Brahman, and so from there we finally reach the last stage—*turiya ga*, "to come into the Fourth (*turiya*)"—and liberation.

You may have noticed something odd at the end of the last sentence, in this view of the stages the seventh and ultimate stage is called the "Fourth." Here again we have an example of the symbolic message of the number four, which expresses "completion, perfection, and order."

▸ ▸ BEHIND THE NUMBERS

The Fourth and the "X + 1 Syndrome"

Indian culture, as we've amply seen, has a tendency to classify objects, institutions, and knowledge and, once these are established, often advances a category that transcends whatever's been classified. This category represents a more perfect condition than those in the original classification. This is what Patrick Olivelle calls the "X + 1 syndrome." He notes it happens frequently in sets of four that are made by adding one to the preexisting three.[1]

Some texts then talk about a fifth state that transcends the fourth. It's called *turyatita*, literally "to go beyond (*atita*)" by implication the Fourth. In this state, the "unity consciousness that began in turya is consummated in turyatita in which the whole universe appears as the Self."[2]

▸ ▸ BEHIND THE NUMBERS

Seven in Sanskrit

The Sanskrit word for seven is *saptan* (in compounds prefixing other words, *sapta*). The Sanskrit dictionary tells us that seven is sacred to Hindus. It goes on then to list a grab bag of sevens, while providing no details about any of them: some of them found in our everyday world, others only in the mythic. So there are seven rivers, seven oceans, seven cities, seven divisions of the world, seven ranges of mountains, seven *rishis*, seven sages (*vipras*), seven demons (*danava*), seven horses of the sun, seven flames of fire, and seven sacrificial rites.

◂ ◂

TWO POLES OF YOGA DISCIPLINE: PRACTICE (*ABHYASA*) AND DISPASSION (*VAIRAGYA*)

Practice without dispassion is conducive to an abnormal ego-inflation and hunger for power. . . . Dispassion without practice is like a blunt knife. . . . Both poles need to be cultivated simultaneously and with prudence.

Georg Feuerstein, *The Essence of Yoga*

Like the common household battery, the discipline of yoga has two poles. The positive pole is called *abhyasa*; its negative opposite is *vairagya*. Just as a battery powers a flashlight or TV remote, abhyasa and vairagya power the yogi's efforts toward liberation.

The two poles are introduced in YS 1.12, where they're recommended for quieting the fluctuations of consciousness, the central goal of Patanjali's teaching.[3] I checked with about 15 different translations of the text to see how the most experienced and knowledgeable translators—Georg Feuerstein, Edwin Bryant, and James Woods among them—rendered our two words into English.

All of our translators agreed that *practice* is the best English word for *abhyasa*. For Patanjali, of course, practice meant the eight limbs (*ashta anga*) covered over the second half of the text's second chapter and the first few sutras of chapter three, or possibly the three limbs of Kriya Yoga covered very briefly at YS 2.1–2. Now the English term *practice* certainly gets the idea of Sanskrit *abhyasa* across to non-Sanskritists, but as is common with many Sanskrit words, one English word doesn't quite relay abhyasa's full impact. Let's take a closer look and see if there are other meanings associated with the word that might expand on the idea of practice.

We'll start by separating the prefix *abhi-* from the root word, *as* (the *i* at the end of *abhi-* turns into a *y* when it's connected to the leading *a* of the root). *Abhi-* expresses the notion of going toward or into. Toward or into what? The root word, *as*.

Now we English speakers might be fooled by *as*. After all, how much meaning can be packed into two letters? Since this is Sanskrit, the answer is a lot. Look closely at the word. Does it remind you of any other Sanskrit word? Indeed, *asana*. Nowadays we think of *asana* as a pose or posture, but these aren't really strict translations. If we look *as* up in the Sanskrit dictionary, we find the leading definition is "to sit."

Originally an asana was a low platform on which yogis sat for their daily meditation. Then over time the word shifted to include the sitting position itself. Don't forget that initially for Patanjali, an asana was nothing other than a seated position like Lotus (*padmasana*) or Hero (*virasana*). We have to wait maybe a thousand years before nonseated asanas become prevalent in Hatha Yoga.

What else can we learn from *as*? Returning to the dictionary, we see it also means both "to be present" and "to do anything without interruption." Here are two more pieces of information pertinent to our practice. What does it mean to be present? Obviously, we're always physically present when we practice, but what about mentally? Have you ever done a practice and then, when finished, feel like you weren't really "there" most of the time? To be present means to make a concerted effort to stay fully conscious of whatever we're doing and thinking and feeling in our practice and not allow our attention to drift away from that self-focus.

It's also important to note this presence might be compared to what's called a "fair witness." This is an individual trained to objectively observe what's taking place in front of them without making subjective comments or assessments. The Indian sage J. Krishnamurti called this kind of observation "choiceless awareness."[4] As we maintain our presence, we should also be persistent; that is, we should stay with our daily practice through all the inevitable highs and lows, successes and failures. Persistence builds momentum, which makes it easier to maintain a daily practice over time.

There's one more meaning that *as* brings to both *asana* and *abhyasa*. I feel it's as essential to practice as being present and persevering, and that's "to celebrate." This urges us to treat each practice as a joyful acknowledgment of our life in yoga, then of course take that out into the world and spread it around freely.

The 15 translations of *vairagya* weren't in as complete agreement as they were for abhyasa, but two words emerged as English favorites, *dispassion* and *detachment* (or nonattachment). With these two words, we come face-to-face with two of the major efforts of Patanjali's system: to diligently purge ourselves of any and all attachment we have to both the inner and outer worlds to prepare ourselves for meditation and to withdraw from matter to prepare for the ultimate and final withdrawal to aloneness (*kaivalya*).

We can all agree the essential ingredients of abhyasa—to persevere in, to be present to, and to celebrate our practice—contribute to our yoga success. It's indeed the positive pole of the battery and should involve a letting go, but only of destructive emotions and desires. To purge ourselves of human emotions and reject the material world isn't why we practice yoga in the twenty-first century. Let's see if we can find an alternative way to understand vairagya.

We'll start, as we did with abhyasa, by taking the root of *vairagya*, which is *ranj*, "to be dyed or colored," and to be variously "excited, glad, charmed, delighted, enamoured." We have to wonder who wouldn't be pleased to be dyed in this way? The answer is Patanjali. If we prefix *ranj* with *vi-*, which expresses "division," we get *vairagya*, a word which means "growing pale." With Patanjali's practice, all of our dye is washed away. It makes for a fascinating image. Our likes and dislikes color us, and the more obsessively we hold on to them, the more our consciousness is colored by them.

But if we can step away from our desires—or more precisely, from the stranglehold they have on our mind and the appeal they have to our ego—then we can live with desire but not be dominated by it. As the color of our desire fades from consciousness, we become more and more transparent, and the light of the Absolute shines in and through us.

▸ ▸ STORY

The Kitten and the Monkey

Abhyasa and vairagya are by themselves each a path of yoga. The former is called the path of the Monkey, who as a baby, must hold on tightly to its mother's back when transported so as not to fall. This way to liberation depends on both the grace of the deity and the yogi's own effort. It's also known as the Northern school.

The latter is the path of the Kitten. She's carried in the grip of her mother's jaws, secured there by the scruff of her neck. Unlike the Monkey, the Kitten makes no effort whatsoever and is entirely dependent on the grace of the deity to transport her to her ultimate destination. This way to liberation depends entirely on that grace and is also known as the Southern school.

◂ ◂

EIGHT LIMBS (*ANGA*)

Restraint (*yama*), voluntary penance (*niyama*), seat (*asana*), breath restraint (*pranayama*), sense withdrawal (*pratyahara*), concentration (*dharana*), meditation (*dhyana*), *samadhi* are the eight limbs of yoga.

Yoga Sutra 2.29

Because the *Yoga Sutra* is so widely read, especially in teacher training programs, quite often when we come across certain numbers between one and 10—notably five and eight—they ring a bell with something we've studied in the text. Five naturally suggests the yamas and niyamas (see pp. 107 and 108), and to a lesser degree the fluctuations (*vritti*), and the afflictions (*klesha*, see p. 119).

But eight might be the better example, because it inevitably recalls Patanjali's original, well-known eight-limb (*ashtanga*) discipline.[5] This raises the question: how many limbs are needed to comprise an effective practice? *The Dictionary of All Scriptures* credits seven as a number signifying "completion or consummation," indicating the "beginning and ending of a cycle."[6] Patanjali's eighth limb, samadhi, does precisely what the quote claims for it: it opens an "entrance into a new state or condition of the soul."[7]

While many subsequent schools followed suit with eight limbs, not all of them did. Most of the schools with fewer than eight have six, though there's one text I found with a five-limb setup.

It's in the *Vayu Purana* and called Pashupata or Maheshvara Yoga.[8] We're told it's been "proclaimed by Rudra," which as we know is another name for Shiva. Many traditional texts are attributed to divine sources, which imbues them with a special prestige. Oddly, the practices here are called *dharmas*, which suggests their performance aligns the yogi with the universal order (see p. 130). The five are pranayama, dhyana, pratyahara, dharana, and smarana, which means "recollection," that is, of the yogi's deity of choice with bhakti-like devotion.

Two things stand out about this arrangement. First is the unusual order of the limbs, at least compared to the logical progression of limbs in the Yoga Sutra. Second, as is fairly common in Hatha texts, there aren't any formal lists of yamas and niyamas. There are 10 in all, a few of which are a bit out of the ordinary and so worth listing: knowledge (*jnana*), nonattachment (*vairagya*), glorious prosperity, penance (*tapas*), truth (*satya*), forbearance (*kshama*), firmness (*dridha*), creativity, self-comprehension, and dominance.

The six-limb schools are more numerous than the five-limb ones, and they generally fall into one of two categories. One consists of mostly obscure texts (at least to a nonscholar like myself) that make mention of six limbs without detailing them. An example is the MVT, whose translator, Somadeva Vasudeva, assures us that a six-limb system is presented in the text though "without a formal list of these ancillaries (*anga*) or even a statement that their number is six."[9] Vasudeva orders the limbs in a way that, compared to the classical order, at first glance seems jumbled: pranayama, dharana, *tarka* ("reasoning, speculation"), dhyana, samadhi, pratyahara.

Now it turns out, once the limbs are rendered in this way, the MVT belongs to a subcategory of six-limb schools. Rather than get ahead of ourselves, let's hold off until we get to the relevant texts before going into this one.

The *Avadhuta Gita* sort of fits in here but not as we might expect. An *avadhuta* is someone who's "shaken off" all worldly attachments and obligations, so "feels no need of observing any rules, either secular or religious. He seeks nothing, avoids nothing."[10] As a consequence, any and every kind of practice, including yoga, is ultimately dismissed as unnecessary. The Self, writes the author, "certainly does not become pure through the practice of six-limbed yoga," nor through "destruction of the mind," nor by the "instructions of the teacher. It [i.e., the Self] is Itself the Truth, It is Itself the illumined One."[11]

In the second category are texts that name the six limbs, and these can be further divided into two subcategories. In one, the texts take

Patanjali's eight limbs and omit yama and niyama; these six-limbers include the *Dhyana Bindu Upanishad* (DBU), the YCU, and the *Goraksha Shatakam* (GSh).[12] The second subgroup takes the truncated six and substitutes tarka for asana. Texts in this subgroup include, as previously noted, the MVT, the *Maitri Upanishad* (MaiU) and *Amrita Nada Upanishad*.[13]

There's one significant Hatha text, the aforementioned GS, that has seven limbs, which up front aren't named by the practices themselves; rather, each limb is first designated by the expected benefit of the associated practice, which is then described in the body of the text.[14] So the limbs are purification (*shodhana*), which is accomplished through the six acts (*shad karma*, see p. 131); strength (*dridha*) through asana; stability (*sthairya*) through mudra; calmness (*dhairya*) through pratyahara; lightness (*laghava*) through pranayama; perception (*pratyaksha*), that is, of the Self, through meditation; and undefiled-ness (*nirlipta*), that is, liberation, through samadhi.

As I mentioned at the start, there's one text—the *Tejo Bindu Upanishad*—that has a 15-limb practice (*panca dasha anga yoga*). All of Patanjali's eight limbs are included in the 15 in their classical order (as limbs 1, 2, 7, 11, 12, 13, 14, 15), supplemented by seven limbs.

1. Yama is the control of the "manifold senses" in and through the knowledge that "all is the Brahman."
2. Niyama is the complete inward turn of consciousness, which brings "exquisite pleasure."
3. Tyaga is the renunciation of the "phenomenal world," capable of giving the yogi "instantaneous liberation from bondage."
4. Quiescence or silence (*mauna*) results from the impossibility to "speak of That, from which speech returns."
5. Proper place (*desha*) for practice, one that's totally isolated from other people.
6. Proper time (*kala*, spelled with a long first *a* and is pronounced KAH-luh) is obtaining "with the twinkling of the eye as the unit," of the "peerless immeasurable expanse of Bliss."

7. Siddhasana is reaching the "final attainment," Brahman.

8. Mula bandha is here the restraint of the mind.

9. Bodily equilibrium (*deha samya*) among the three bodies (gross, subtle and causal) enables "their dissolution in the well-poised Brahman."

10. Stability of introspection (*drk sthiti*) is introspection replete with wisdom, through which the yogi looks "upon the world as filled with the Brahman."

11. Pranayama is the "suppression of all vital function."

12. Pratyahara is the "pleasant experience" when the mind finds the Atman in the objects of desire.

13. Dharana is the "state of abstraction attained by the mind, when it sees the Brahman whithersoever it might traverse."

14. Dhyana is the "state which rests on no support, but the real devotion to the attitude, 'I am only the Brahman,'" which "yields exquisite pleasure."

15. Samadhi is the steady mind of the "form of the Brahman."[15]

‣ ‣ BEHIND THE NUMBERS

Eight Allegorical Limbs

Typically, when we think of a limb (*anga*), there's at least one, sometimes two or more, practices associated with it. But there are a few descriptions of limbs scattered here and there in the literature in which one or more of the limbs are allegorical or, if you prefer, symbolic.

One of the best examples takes up about half of the very short (one printed page) *Laghu Avadhuta Upanishad*. It tells us that: detachment from the physical body and five senses is yama; unwavering attachment to the highest truth is niyama; indifference toward all things is asana; the firm belief this whole world is false is pranayama; focusing the mind into itself is pratyahara; maintaining a steadfast mind is concentration; the thought "I am only pure consciousness" is meditation; and the total oblivion of meditation is samadhi.

The advantage of this allegory is that we don't need to be sequestered to do our practice (if that practice is based on the classical model), we can practice just about anywhere with, of course, some reasonable restrictions; for example, "total oblivion" wouldn't be appropriate when driving on the freeway at 65 mph, or even on city streets at 25 mph for that matter. But surely, at select times during our day as we go about our business (no matter what our practice model is), we could "step aside" from what we're doing and spend a few minutes with the thought, "I am only pure consciousness."

▸ ▸ BEHIND THE NUMBERS

Eight in Sanskrit

The Sanskrit word for eight is *ashtan* (in compounds prefixing other words, *ashta*). The yogis know eight ways (*ashta dharma marga*) of reaching liberation (*moksha*): sacrifice (*yaga*), constant repetition of the hymns of the Veda or OM (*vedabhyasa*), charity (*dana*), asceticism (*tapas*), truthfulness (*satya*), patience (*shama*), compassion (*daya*), and lack of desire. This last way is rather confusing. Don't we need desire to urge us toward liberation? Isn't this what the Vedantins call mumukshu? This reminds me of a statement by Abhinavagupta, who prescribes in yoga what is called a "perfectly relaxed way of life." He says, "Do not reject and do not accept; enjoy everything as it is." He also says, "Do not leave anything, do not take anything; be in yourself (the Self) and enjoy everything as it is."[16]

To reach liberation, we need correct knowledge, and there are eight ways to obtain this: direct perception (*pratyasha*), inference (*anumana*), analogy (*upamana*), testimony (*shabda*), presumption (*arthapatti*), nonrecognition (*anupalabdhi*), reason (*sambhava*), and tradition (*aitihya*).

Of these eight, nonrecognition is a bit odd. Anupalabdhi is the way we apprehend an absence. "When all the conditions for the perception of *x* are present, and yet *x* is not perceived, in that case this non-perception would lead to a true cognition of the absence of *x*."[17]

In plain English, if it's possible for us to see something and we see nothing, then we can say quite truly that we saw something wasn't there.

On the other side, the yogis know eight ways of suffering (*ashta kashta*): lust (*kama*), anger (*krodha*), greed (*lobha*), delusion (*moha*), arrogance (*mada*), rivalry (*matsarya*), pride (*dambha*), and jealousy (*asuya*).

◂ ◂

10 SELF-RESTRAINTS (*YAMA*)

For a living being, practice of . . . yoga cannot be had without these two (*yama* and *niyama*). . . . The practitioners of hatha can attain *satva* through *yama* and *niyama*.

Sundaradeva, *Hatha Tatva Kaumudi* 6.8

Because of the popularity of the YS, there are two numbers fixed in many students minds' in regard to the limbs of practice and the self-restraints (*yama*) and observances (*niyama*): eight for the limbs and five for the latter two. While eight-limb practices are common, there are also texts that offer practices with six, or seven, or even 15 limbs for a general yoga practice and 16 in Mantra Yoga.

We also find the yama and niyama pentads in the YS aren't carved in stone, regarding both number and content. Five, as we've speculated, is a popular number for lists because we can associate each item in the list with one of our digits as a memory aid, so that I'm nonviolent with my thumb, for example, truthful with my index finger, and so on. Then what's true of one hand is doubly true of two, and indeed we find in Hatha texts that the yamas and niyamas are usually—but not always—doubled from five to 10.

The texts with 10 yamas usually include four of Patanjali's: nonviolence, truthfulness, no stealing, and celibacy; for some reason "greedlessness" (*aparigraha*) is left out, and cleanliness or purity (*shauca*)—one of Patanjali's niyamas—is shifted to a yama. The *Shandilya Upanishad* (SU), by the way, divides cleanliness into two kinds: external and internal. The latter implies "purity of mind" which is "attained through study of (spiritual) lore" on Atman. The former is done with "earth and water," in other words, by bathing, which then can be counted among the niyamas, emphasizing again its importance.[18]

Three of the remaining five yamas present the translator—or at least this translator—with a bit of a problem. Sanskrit is multivalent, which means many of its words have various meanings; the one that's finally settled on is determined by the context. The easy two are moderate diet (*mitahara*) and compassion (*anukampa*). The former reflects the Hatha yogi's concern about what food to eat, described at length, for example, in GS 5.16–30. The opening verse warns if we start yoga practice without a "measured (*mita*) diet (*ahara*)," we risk getting several unnamed diseases and our practice will fail. Diet doesn't seem to concern Patanjali, but although compassion isn't among his yamas, Patanjali does encourage it as a fitting response to others' sorrow.[19]

Then we have three Sanskrit words—*arjava, kshama, dhriti*—that could head off in any number of translation directions. So instead of me just choosing one, I'll list all reasonable possibilities and let you decide which works best for you (I'll put in **bold** the translations from the texts):

- *arjava* (rectitude, propriety of act or observance; honesty, frankness, sincerity, **straightforwardness**)
- *kshama* (patience, forbearance, indulgence; have patience or bear with, **forgiveness**)
- *dhriti* (firmness, constancy, **fortitude**)

10 OBSERVANCES (*NIYAMA*)

Niyama is the continuous application (of Consciousness in its entirety) to intrinsic categories and the rejection (by it) of extrinsic categories. Exquisite pleasure is attained by the wise man, through Niyama.

Tejo Bindu Upanishad 1.18

Here we see again that the 10 niyamas of the Hatha list are built on the foundation of four of five of Patanjali's niyamas—recall that cleanliness has been shifted to the yamas. They are (with Patanjali's equivalent following in parentheses): contentment or joy (*santosha*), austerity (*tapas*), listening to scriptural and saintly doctrines (*svadhyaya*), belief in God (*ishvara pranidhana*).

The remaining six niyamas are worship of something greater than the Self (e.g., God), generosity (*dana*), modesty (*lajja*), shame or modesty (*hri*), recitation of mantras (*japa*), and "constancy in the observance of the injunctions and prohibitions laid down in the Veda" (*vrata*).[20]

▸ ▸ BEHIND THE NUMBERS

Other Yama Lists

We can find other lists of yamas or, though not specifically labeled as such, yama-like behavioral injunctions scattered here and there in Hatha texts. The lists may check in with six items.[21] Svatmarama's six are probably the most useful for us modern students, except maybe "abandoning public contact," which the old yogis believed was harmful in several ways, particularly the powerful influences our culture exerts on us, often without our realization, that helps to keep us locked into our limited egoic identity.

I made a very informal survey for yamas-niyamas in the texts I have access to and found over 160 listed. I won't include them all here; instead, I'll list the 10 I feel are most useful for modern students (in alphabetical order): celebration (including joyfulness, wonder, and curiosity), compassion, courage (including determination), even-mindedness (avoidance of extreme emotions like anger, greed), faith, generosity, modesty, self-study (including listening to all doctrines and the desire for Self-liberation), truthfulness, and finally—out of order because I think it's the most important—desire for the good of the world (*hita iccha*, including service).

◂ ◂

10 in Sanskrit

The Sanskrit word for 10 is *dashan* (in compounds prefixing other words, *dasha*).

In old India, there were mendicants called *parivragakas*, literally "to go about" (*pari*) "wandering" (*vraga*), who roamed country to spread the "ideas or truths which they had derived from the sacred scriptures, in the light of which they had tried to reorder their own lives."[22]

In time the philosopher Shankara organized the Order of 10 Names (*dashanamin*), and the mendicants who joined were required to forsake their caste names and were given new names ending in one of 10 surnames: *tirtha* ("ford," the confluence of three rivers, "signifying bathing in the rivers of knowledge and truth"), *ashrama* ("hermitage," free from the "bonds of mundane existence"), *vana* ("forest"), *aranya* ("forest," a person who finds "bliss in doing penance in the forest"), *giri* ("mountain," a person as "serene and steady as a mountain"), *parvata* ("mountain," living in retreat at the "foot of a mountain possessing the knowledge of transience"), *sagara* ("ocean," a person who understands the "ocean of truth"), *sarasvati* (the name of the mythic river and the goddess of learning, "perfect knowledge"), *bharati* ("eloquence," filled with knowledge), and *puri* ("city," in "constant union" with the supreme soul).[23] (For more on tirtha and sarasvati, see p. 78.) The wanderers were supposed to keep moving always, and in extreme cases, "not even a roof over their head except the sky."[24]

◂ ◂

SIX CLEANSING ACTS (*KARMA*)

It's typical for a traditional yoga practice to begin with a period of behavioral self-purification in regard to both self and others. This preparation might include practices to instill valued behaviors (nonviolence, truthfulness), to clean out the physical body with certain austerities (*tapas*), to inspire the mind by reading spiritually oriented texts (*svadhyaya*), and to pay homage to the deity and let it know you're now open to its presence (*ishvara pranidhana*).

Among modern teachers, it's generally agreed that these practices—usually collected under the headings yama and niyama, as the first two limbs of Patanjali's eight-limb practice—are the basics of a yoga practice. B.K.S. Iyengar writes, "In order to fly, a bird needs two wings. Similarly, to climb the ladder of spiritual wisdom, the ethical and mental disciplines are essential."[25] We can look at these two limbs as a kind of cleansing practice in relation to others (*yama*) and ourselves (*niyama*) before tackling the next six limbs.

But not the GS: its purificatory preparation takes up most of the first chapter, and its practices are strictly physical.[26] Here we see one of the many differences between Patanjali Yoga and Hatha Yoga, or what Gheranda calls the "yoga of the pot" (*Ghatastha Yoga*)—the pot being the physical body. Patanjali's arena is consciousness (*citta*) and the separation of the Self from matter, while Gerandha's focus is the body and the awakening of the goddess Kundalini.

By all accounts this event releases a lightning-like bolt of energy up along the spine. Gopi Krishna, in a well-known account of his Kundalini awakening, for which he was completely unprepared, describes the "stream of liquid light" that, "with a roar like that of a waterfall," entered his brain through his spinal cord.[27] For months he suffered through terrible physical pain and depression until he was able to find the help he needed to understand what had happened to him and make peace with the goddess.

The collection of Gheranda's practices together is called the "six acts" (*shat karma*), but this is something of a misnomer. Three of the six are themselves collections of acts, so there are 21 acts in all. There's no adequate English translation for three of the six categories, which are (the number of exercises in each category follow in parentheses): washing (*dhauti*, 13), "bladder" (*basti* or *vasti*, 2), neti (1), *nauli* (1), *trataka* (1), and "skull brightener" (*kapalabhati*, 3). Again, the first step to spiritual wisdom involves a purification, but this one is strictly physical rather than psychological.

I don't think it's necessary to say much about these practices. We already do a few of them for our general hygiene: we routinely brush our teeth and clean our tongue and ears. A few others shouldn't be performed unless we're under the immediate and closely watched supervision of a Self-realized teacher. These karmas include lengthening our tongue by first severing the frenum, the flap of skin that connects the tongue to the floor of the mouth. Then we're supposed to methodically pull and stretch the tongue day by day to ready ourselves for *khecari mudra*, the "moving in space" seal. Or there's something called "purify the root" (*mula shodhana*), which would have us, apparently, draw our intestines out of our body through the anus, and wash them out in a river.

Just briefly then, some of the acts involve passing water through the alimentary canal, self-induced vomiting, "flossing" the nasal passages with a thread inserted through one nostril and pulled out through the mouth, and swallowing a long, thin cloth, then rhythmically churning the abdominal muscles to swab the stomach. One of them, "skull brightener" (*kapalabhati*), in which the lower abdominal muscles are repeatedly and quickly contracted to exhale and released to receive the inhale on the rebound, may be familiar to you.

The karmas actually might not even be needed. Svatmarama says that only those students with excess fat and phlegm need to do these exercises.[28] If neither of these affect us, we're free to skip over this part of the practice. The anonymous author twice states that these practices should be kept secret. This obsession for secrecy is common throughout all the limbs of Hatha Yoga. The claim is that secrecy preserves the practice's potency,[29] revealing them to outsiders and the noninitiated strips them of their powers. The problem then, as you can see, is that the publication of these translations reveals these secrets, at least superficially, to countless noninitiates. Are we to assume that because of this, traditional Hatha Yoga's cat is way out of the bag and any transformational kick it once had is now forever lost?

What are the results of these practices according to the anonymous author of the GS? Like many other kinds of practices, the karmas are said to destroy disease—of the stomach and intestines, heart, and skin, among others—clear disorders of phlegm and bile, stave off old age and death, give the yogi vision and hearing at a distance (clairvoyance and clairaudience), and a godlike body (*devadeha*). All those critics of modern yoga who condemn it for being too physically oriented, too concerned with body image, please take note. While we often picture yogis as underweight skeletons dressed in rags, at least this one text suggests yogis could have a "body beautiful." There's a precedent for this that goes back at least 300 years, though it's true enough that we may have taken the physical too far and cut ourselves off from the central spiritual thrust. But it's hard to ignore the promise that with water *vasti*, our body becomes like that of Kama, the Hindu Cupid.[30]

▸ ▸ PRACTICE

Skull Cleansing (Kapala Randhra Dhauti)

Here's a simple exercise from the GS that to me helps quiet the brain before shavasana and bedtime.[31] The text specifies using the right thumb, but this is simply another example, common in the old texts—and in fact all over the world—of right-handism. So if you're left-handed, I encourage you to use that hand.

Touch your thumb to the space between the eyebrows at the bridge of the nose and gently rub. The text doesn't specify how to rub, up and down or circularly, so experiment with both. According to Gheranda, this purifies the nadis (and presumably the triveni, see p. 76) and induces *divya drishti*, "divine sight." It's recommended this be done just after waking, after meals, and before bedtime.

I should mention there's a bit of an issue with this practice. I have seven translations of the GS, but only three describe it as a thumb massage for the nose bridge. Three others interpret *bhalarandhra* as the "aperture at the roof of the mouth" (translation by James Mallinson) or the "hindmost part of the roof of the mouth" (translation from Kaivalyadhama), which I take to be the soft palate.

And what about the seventh translation? This one is done by some-one named Shyam Ghosh, who instructs us to massage the "soft parts (sides) of the forehead . . . with the right thumb."[32]

◂ ◂

PRACTICE TIME: THE THREE, FOUR, OR FIVE JUNCTIONS (*SANDHYA*)

That knower of the Brahman, who draws in vital air during the period of the junctions and drinks it, in the course of three months, his speech becomes erudite and blessed.

Shandilya Upanishad 1.7.46

I think most of us are happy if we can get one yoga practice in each day. The old yogis, however, had no job, no families; the main focus of their lives was yoga. Depending on the teaching they were following, they were enjoined to practice three, four, or five times each day, and these times were determined by the sun's journey across the sky.

According to the Indian tradition, there are at least two stretches of time in every day when practice is especially propitious: sunrise and sun-set. Because these are times when light and dark are blended, they're also called *sandhyas*. The Sanskrit-English dictionary suggests the word "may be connected with" *sam*, "complete," and *dhyai*, "meditation." In other words, these junctions are the perfect times for practice and meditation. Why is this?

All humans past and present, regardless of age, gender, and social status or where in the world they are, experience the same life-shaping forces, such as gravity and the alternation of light and dark. This external back-and-forth, the yogis say, influences our internal forces of dark and light, symbolized by the lunar ida nadi and the solar pingala nadi. Gener-ally, one of these two nadis dominates the other—and we can feel this as one nostril being more open than the other—and this domination shifts back and forth between the two every hour or so. But there are times when the two forces join in the middle, in the central sushumna nadi, and that is the "period known as sandhya... the real sandhya is when the pranas start to flow in sushumna."[33]

According to *The Daily Practice of the Hindus*, the morning sandhya readies us to enter upon our "worldly duties" and should start before the sun rises and finish with the "rising of the Sun." The evening sandhya, which ends our day after completing our duties, should start before the sun begins to set and finish "with the complete setting of that luminary and the rising of the stars."[34]

The SS recommends four practice sessions every day, at four significant sandhya: sunrise, noon, sunset, and midnight. Each session should consist of 20 rounds of the preliminary breathing practice known as the "purification of the nadis" (*nadi shodhana*). There are no specific timings noted in the text for the inhales, exhales, and retentions. All that's said is that the inhales and exhales should be done "gently, not quickly,"[35] and that we should retain the breath for as long as we can.[36] Out of curiosity, I followed these instructions as best I could to find out how long a single practice session might last. I timed one round with no retention after the exhale at about 45 seconds. Multiplying this number by 20 and then dividing the product by 60 yielded a session of about 15 minutes, though it's possible an experienced yogi will take somewhat more time for each round.

The HYP agrees that we should practice four times a day at those junctions, but ups the number of rounds in each session to 80,[37] which quadruples the number of rounds suggested by the SS. Logically, this will also quadruple the time it takes to complete one practice session; in other words, if 20 rounds are estimated to take 15 minutes, 80 will take at least an hour.

The GS first suggests practicing eight times a day, every three hours,[38] which feels extreme even for traditional yoga. The anonymous author of the text immediately reduces that number first to five times daily, at morning, noon, evening, midnight, and the "fourth" (*catur thaka*), presumably around 4 a.m., and then to three, at morning, noon, and 8 p.m. Though he's very detailed about how long the breath should be inhaled (16 counts), exhaled (32 counts), and retained (64 counts), he says nothing about how many rounds make up each practice session. One round, however, will probably take a little more than two minutes, so 20 rounds will take about 40 minutes, and 80 rounds an impractical 2½ hours.

8

STAGES AND OBSTACLES
BY THE NUMBERS

When Samadhi is being practised, obstacles
forcibly make their appearance.

Tejo Bindu Upanishad 1.40

In his commentary on *Yoga Sutra* 1.1, Vyasa outlines five stages (*bhumi*)
of consciousness (*citta*), or at least what he thinks of as five. These are
scattered (*kshipta*), stupefied or dull (*mudha*), agitated (*vikshipta*), one-
pointed (*ekagra*), and restricted (*niruddha*). Ordered lists of this kind,
very often with five, six, or seven items, are common in the yoga tradition. They often serve as road maps from starting point *A* to the destination at point *B*, helping yogis orient themselves in the general scheme of
the practice. We can see such a process in Patanjali's eight limbs, through
which the yogi gradually withdraws from public interaction governed by
the yamas and niyamas to the self-imposed isolation from the public in
the second four stages.

There's a slight problem though with designating the five items on
this list as "stages," which is an accurate translation of the Sanskrit *bhumi*.
We expect something in stages to be hierarchical, leading us step-by-step
from a less desirable place or situation to a more desirable place or situation. But if we look carefully at the first two stages, it's apparent they're

not hierarchical, but rather head and tail of the same coin. That said, we'll continue to talk about five stages to avoid confusion.

Stages have to be based on something—usually something that's getting better as the stages advance (though sometimes worse) and has some appealing goal or satisfying resolution. The stages here are based on the purposeful, progressive stilling of our normally lively consciousness, the proximate goal being its complete quiescence.

Kshipta and mudha bookend the range of human emotions. Kshipta is ruled by rajas guna (see p. 36), and when in its thrall, we're racked by Category 5 storms that blow and rage (and crack their cheeks, as King Lear would have it). When mudha is dominant, tamas takes over, and we sink into a Kierkegaardian existential ennui. We've all experienced these extremes and most everything in between.

Of the five, kshipta and mudha are the obstacle stages we know best and in which we have the most interest. Does Vyasa have some words of wisdom that will help us get a handle on this pair and everything in between? Maybe then if we work at it, we can graduate to stage three. But here Vyasa reminds us indirectly that texts like the YS were compiled primarily for yogis who have dedicated their lives to the practice and not average folks like us. These two stages are judged to be outside the pale of yoga, so he skips past them with barely a mention.

We see the name of the third stage, vikshipta, is very close to that of the first, but with a *vi-* prefix, which I take to mean "away from"; in other words, in this stage we're moving away from the first two stages and, with dedication and a little luck, transitioning to the next two yoga-related stages. In vikshipta, rajas still dominates but now some sattva is becoming evident. The "concentration attainable," as Vyasa describes it, is "subordinated to the moments of unrest."[1] We're still not card-carrying yogis, but we're getting closer. We find ourselves in a tug-of-war between the two stages we're trying to leave behind and the two we see ahead of us, if still only vaguely.

With the final two stages, ekagra and niruddha, we enter yoga practice proper. Vyasa explains that consciousness is one-pointed when it slows down and is consistently engaged with a single thought. The rajas/sattva imbalance of the previous stage has now flipped over: sattva dominates, though still roiled occasionally by rajas. I assume accomplished meditators have some direct experience with the fourth stage, though many of us have unknowingly entered in at random times in our lives. When were you last totally absorbed in a book, film, or project at work—one that held and focused your attention on a single thought, until some outside distraction broke the spell? That was the fourth, or an approximation of the stage since it wasn't induced purposely by practice. The fourth is said to "weaken the kleshas, loosen the bonds of karma,"[2] and pry open the door to the fifth.

By the way, ekagra isn't limited to humans. Watch how dogs sit steady and comfortable in *Shvanasana* (Dog Pose) and focus their attention laser-like on something their human companions might be eating.

We might imagine the fifth stage, now suffused with pure sattva, "when all the modifications (*vritti*) have come under control (*nirodha*)," is accessible only to those rare individuals with the superhuman persistence and courage to take the last step successfully. This is true to a certain extent. But the fact is, as Vyasa reveals much to our surprise, this stage, known also as unconscious (*asamprajnata*) samadhi, is a "universal attribute of the mind-field (*citta*), common to all levels."[3] In other words, all of us are, right now, in samadhi, though maybe not in the way we might imagine.

FIVE AFFLICTIONS (*KLESHA*)

Pleasure is only a fleeting interlude in a panorama of suffering.
Benjamin Walker, "Suffering," *The Hindu World*

The origin of the rather disturbing quote, "Life is hard and then you die," is a matter lively debate. While I'm sure we can't attribute it to Patanjali, still and all, the sentiment isn't far off from his view of embodied existence, except he might add, "and then you're born again . . . and again . . . and again, and each time is more of the same." There's nothing we can do about all the suffering we've gone through in the countless lives we've lived before—that's suffering under the bridge—but we can do something about the suffering we're assured of in future lives. What's that? Have a look at the YS.

The cause of all this unhappiness is the five *kleshas*, a word that sums up how Patanjali rates our situation in life: "pain, affliction, distress, anguish, hardship, trouble." There's more, but you get the picture. The source of this unpleasant and, no doubt many people would say, mostly undeserved suffering is something called *avidya*, literally "not-knowing." There are actually two ways to spell and so pronounce this word, one with a short final *a*, pronounced uh-VID-yuh, the other with a long final *a*, pronounced uh-vid-YAH. The former refers to everyday ignorance, "unwise, foolish"; the latter refers to spiritual ignorance. It's very possible to be possessed by the long-*a avidya*, and yet be quite brilliant in the everyday world, though I'm not sure the reverse would be true.

Avidya is a generalized "not-knowing," an across-the-board confusion really, of the transient with the eternal, of the impure with the pure, of misery with happiness, and the not-self with the Self.[4] In other words, there's only one thing we can say about the world and ourselves with any confidence, and that is, we don't know. What's worse, I suppose, though superficially it might make it more bearable, is that many of us don't know that we don't know, a double whammy.

What is it we don't know? We don't know that our basic assumptions about ourselves and the world are somewhat to sorely mistaken. As Patanjali puts it (here I paraphrase), believing the transient to be eternal, the impure (i.e., all matter) to be pure, misery (i.e., our everyday lives) to be happiness, and the not-self (i.e., our ego) to be the Self, is avidya. I especially like James Woods's interpretation of *avidya* as "undifferentiated consciousness."[5]

It's a bizarre and frightening thought. On the surface, everything seems normal—or as normal as is possible in the strange times in which we live—but underneath all the normalcy, we have a vague sensation something is amiss. That gnawing feeling we experience now and again that there's something wrong in our life but we can't quite put a finger on it? That could be avidya, unless we forgot to pay our taxes on time. It only gets worse when we realize all the people around us, especially those we're closest to, are in the same boat. Not only don't we know ourselves; we really don't know anybody else.

Now we might think the toll exacted on our lives by avidya would give us reason enough to take up Patanjali Yoga, but there's more. Avidya, says Vyasa, is the field or propagative soil for four equally unpleasant outgrowths, actually foreshadowed by their source's characteristics. They are desire (*raga*), aversion (*dvesha*), I-am-ness or egoism (*asmita*), and tenacity (*abhinivesha*), the full meaning of which we'll get into shortly.

The first two kleshas go hand in hand. Raga is the "hankering after pleasure," which is anathema in Patanjali's world since it leads to attachment.[6] Dvesha, on the other hand, is the "feeling of opposition, mental disinclination, propensity to hurt and anger towards misery or objects producing misery."[7] It seems like an odd mix, these two. We're warned that any attachment to people, things, or ideas we favor leads straight to suffering, but at the same time, nonattachment to people, things, or ideas we don't favor has the same outcome of suffering. Patanjali has us coming and going; we have to wonder what he would say about indifference.

Asmita is the confusion of our material self with our true Self, which seems to me a more particularized version of avidya's general not-self/ Self mix-up.

Now the fifth klesha, abhinivesha, which we've translated as "tenacity," needs some explanation. Tenacity in what way? The answer is hidden in the word itself: *abhi*, "toward," *ni*, an intensifier, and the root, *vish*, "to dwell." Put this all together and it tells us we have a very strong propensity to go "toward dwelling," or as Vyasa puts it, the "firmly established fear of annihilation." He goes on to assure us such is the case not only for humans, including the wise (*vidvam*) among us, but "every creature always has this craving . . . , even worms from their birth."[8]

Let me spell this out in case you're a bit unclear about what's being said here. Question: do you enjoy living? Yes, there are some unpleasant things about living: both those which affect you personally and the broader world around you, up to and including the entire planet. But all things considered and weighed in the balance, being alive is preferable to . . . not being alive, don't you agree? I do, and I'm sure most people do too.

But what Patanjali is saying is abhinivesha—strongly "going toward dwelling" or clinging to life, in other words—is a klesha and an obstacle. This yoga, remember, is focused on withdrawal—from normal human connection, from movement and breathing, from matter itself including, when the time comes of having attained the nosebleed heights of the eighth limb, our material body. From our very limited Self-ignorant perspective, this is what we call death; from the yogis' enlightened view, however, this is kaivalya, "isolation." Such is one of the necessary outcomes of Patanjali's dualism, in which the Self is favored over nature. The practice of modern yoga has moved off in the opposite direction, toward sustaining life in nature, which is coequal with the Self. I suppose we can still practice abhinivesha, but now as a positive force in which clinging is transformed into a deep caring for our dwelling.

NINE OBSTACLES (*ANTARAYA*)

Obstacle: something that stands in the way of or holds up progress.

from Latin *ob-* against + *stare*, to stand

It's difficult to accept, but yoga and obstacles go hand in hand. Why is that? Recall the yogis' goal is Self-realization which is tantamount to Self-perfection. Because we humans are, to a greater or lesser degree, imperfect creatures, everyone, no matter who, begins their yoga career prone to commit certain mistakes, which are obstacles blocking access to the goal. The yogis try to offset their imperfections by regulating their actions, words, and thoughts according to numbered sets of stringent dos and don'ts, like Patanjali's yamas and niyamas. But as we know, old habits die hard—some harder than others—and there's no guarantee that the yogi in the end will enter the Promised Land.

Sanskrit Words for Obstacle: Vighna, Antaraya, Upasarga, Dosha

There are four words that turn up most frequently in traditional literature that mean or suggest an obstacle. The Yoga Upanishads favor the word *vighna*, which in addition to "obstacle" means "impediment, hindrance," and "any difficulty or trouble." Patanjali, in his Yoga Sutra, favors *antaraya*, a word with a pair of slightly different spellings, although they mean essentially the same thing, "impediment, hindrance, obstacle." Two other words occasionally used are *upasarga*, which means "misfortune, trouble," and *dosha*, "deficiency, disadvantage."

◂ ◂

It's not surprising then that the yogis spent a good deal of time investigating and defining the lineaments of all the obstacles they encountered and then devising methods to master them. Here and there in traditional literature we come across lists of obstacles helpfully inserted by them to forewarn and educate the generations to come—though little did they imagine a generation like ours—about what to look for and how to appropriately respond.

As I gathered obstacles from these lists in about a dozen sources for this section, I became more and more surprised at how many there were. By my rough count there are at least 150, and I'm sure I didn't catch them all. I began to wonder if it was safe to get out of bed in the morning, until I ran across the obstacle of lying around in bed. We're doomed if we do, and doomed if we don't. The obstacles run the gamut from the ridiculous to the hellish, from chewing betel to murder and human trafficking. Only the most persistent and courageous yogis had a chance to reach their goal of Self-realization. As Krishna tells Arjuna:

Of thousands of men,
Scarcely anyone strives for perfection;
Even of the striving and perfected,
Scarcely anyone knows Me in truth.[9]

Most of the obstacles I found are well-known to us in the modern West. They're what we might call equal opportunity obstacles, since they make no distinction between yogis and the rest of us. It's fascinating to see how we're still dealing with issues faced by people more than 1,500 years ago living in a culture so completely different from ours. In the end though, when it comes to obstacles, we're all very much alike.

Probably the best known of these obstacle lists is found in the YS.[10] Recall the goal of Patanjali's practice is to still the fluctuations of consciousness (*citta vrtti*), which in turn clears the way to the realization of our true Self. The nine obstacles on the list, as Vyasa points out, "appear together with the fluctuations of the mind-stuff. They aren't found where the aforesaid fluctuations of mind-stuff are not."[11]

For example, the "false views" obstacle (*bhranti darshana*, see below) is the same as the *viparyaya vritti*, which is "misapprehension, mistaking anything to be the reverse or opposite of what it is"[12]; in other words, both are "wrong knowledge." This is why the yogis were so intent on overcoming obstacles, because by so doing they at the same time restricted the accompanying *vrittis*, calming their mind and bringing them one step closer to Self-realization.

Patanjali's nine obstacles are sickness (*vyadhi*), mental dullness (*styana*), doubt (*samshaya*), carelessness (*pramada*), sloth (*alasya*), intemperance (*avirati*), confusion of philosophies or false view (*bhranti darshana*), unobtained stage (*alabdha bhumikatva*), and instability (*anavashitatva*).

Vyadhi is the only truly physical obstacle. It's easy to see why the yoga tradition considers sickness an obstacle since it's certain not many people feel like practicing with a high fever and runny nose.

Styana is a kind of mental paralysis that's both lethargic and fickle. Samshaya is the inability to choose between two opposing actions, opinions, or beliefs. It often afflicts students whose yoga progress in their estimation has slowed down or stopped altogether, diminishing confidence in both their practice and themselves. "Is yoga practice worthwhile," they wonder, "or is it a waste of time and energy?" Pramada is taking action without reflection, particularly on the possible consequences of that action. Alasya is a lack of initiative, a propensity toward inertia because of physical and/or mental heaviness. Avirati is the thirst for or addiction to worldly objects and sensual experience, the exact opposite of renunciation (*vairagya*). Bhranti darshana is doubt's opposite number. It's a view (*darshana*) that's in error (*bhranti*) or a false opinion or impression either about reality or our own achievements.

The last two obstacles of alabdha bhumikatva and anavashitatva center on the inability to reach or, having reached, the inability to maintain a hold on the advanced levels of the practice. To me, these last two seem more like consequences of the first seven than antaraya in their own right.

The Patanjali obstacles are accompanied by four distractions (*vikshepa*) quite familiar to any student who's come face-to-face with one or more obstacles, which is to say most everyone at some point in their yoga career. These distractions are self-explanatory: pain (*duhkha*), depression (*daurmanasya*)—literally "bad" (*du*) "mind" (*manas*)—physical unsteadiness (*anga ejayatva*)—literally "agitated limbs"—and disturbed breathing.

We're often led to believe the obstacles stem from some personal shortcoming, which may indeed be the case. But Patanjali's nine could also be understood as normal human reactions to the buildup of stresses and strains experienced in just about any endeavor or discipline we engage in regularly over extended periods of time. We should leave perfection to the yogis and always strive to do what one of my teachers said when asked about his philosophy: "Always tell the truth," he responded without hesitation, "and don't hurt anybody."

Mainstream Western religion sometimes warns against or expressly forbids its adherents to participate in yoga classes, even if the class is nothing more spiritual than a sequence of asanas. But our religions and yoga have much in common when it comes to obstacles. For example, seven obstacles found in every one of the books I consulted exactly match the Catholic Church's deadly sins: lust, gluttony, greed, sloth, wrath, envy, and pride.

Many of the obstacles are riffs on these seven: dissolution and its opposite number, excessive fasting; stealing, excessive wealth, usury, miserliness, and possessiveness; apathy, negligence, indifference, laziness, and excessive sleep; hatred and anger, misanthropy, impatience, violence and meanness, and cruelty to animals; jealousy and egoism, arrogance, prejudice, ambition, delusion, fashionable clothes, haughtiness, self-righteousness, and perfume. Perfume?

The litany of obstacles goes on and on, leaving the seven deadly ones in the dust. Bragging, chattering, complaining, gossip, slander, and lying. Then there's the sort of existentialist obstacles of depression, despondency, fear and anxiety, confusion and perplexity, grief and sorrow, and don't be fickle, heedless, and capricious; distracted, secretive, and faithless.

Possibly the strangest obstacle I came across is death. At first glance, I thought it was fairly obvious that being dead would put a serious crimp in the yogis' practice. But then I realized it wasn't *being* dead that's the obstacle, but the *prospect* of being dead. Of course, death affects everyone, not only yogis. We all want to accomplish certain things in our lives, and I'm sure it happens often enough that a person's life project is interrupted midstream by their unexpected demise. The question then is: if the deceased had known the day of their death six months prior, would that have encouraged them to expedite their work on the project and complete it before their leaving?

The yogis' project is obviously Self-realization, but there's another way of looking at it. Not only does the yogi want something, they also want to *avoid* something: and that's rebirth, which for yogis like Patanjali and his school is an unwanted return to the suffering of life. So the yogis want to achieve Self-realization as quickly as possible. If they had some way of predicting their death day, then they would know exactly how quick quickly has to be.

Could the yogis predict when they were going to die? The rational part of my brain emphatically cries, "No!" But the yoga part of my brain, while it doesn't say yes exactly, is willing to suspend disbelief enough to allow, "Who knows? Maybe." It's beyond the scope of this book to go into detail on this subject.

So briefly, Patanjali hints at a pair of death-foretelling meditation techniques in his third chapter. Both are typically incomprehensible to anyone without the necessary consciousness level, even if their sutras are accompanied by an expert commentary. The first technique gives the yogi knowledge of past and future events[13]; the second is more specific: with it we can acquire "knowledge of death."[14]

There are other ways to learn of this. For example, the TBU has an entire section on death-day prediction.[15] I'm sure what's going on here is a lot subtler than it seems on the surface, but the method somehow involves focused breathing, a "well-controlled mind," and knowledge regarding the "cessation of throbbing of his own limbs."

What does that mean? If the throbbing stops in our wrists and ankles, we'll live six months more. If the same occurs in our elbows, we're down to three months, if the armpits, just one month, the belly, 10 days, which is halved if we see a firefly-like radiance. Lastly, if we see some undefined flame, we know we better hurry up, because we only have two days left. So the anonymous author urges us, if we've experienced any of these portents which shorten life, to apply ourselves "to the attainment of final beatitude, resort to silent prayer and meditation and attain the form of the transcendent Atman."

There are also obstacles I call "grumpy yogi obstacles," that purposely drain all the fun and interest out of life to make it easier for them to maintain a strict asceticism. Modern yoga, which is a fully engaged celebration of life, no longer has need of them, and they should be formally retired and laid to rest. An obstacle I haven't mentioned yet is joy, which one list condemns as a great hindrance to realization. As we all now know, joy is one of the emotions that vitalizes our practice and makes life worth living. We can also remove from the obstacles list dancing and singing and musical instruments (flutes and lutes and drums are singled out—sorry, Ringo), excitement, fame and heroism, mouth kissing and passion, scholarship, traveling, joking, and children (maybe after they go off to college).

Nine in Sanskrit

The Sanskrit word for nine is *navan* (in compounds prefixing other words, *nava*). Patanjali lists nine obstacles (*antaraya*) to yoga practice, but only eight ways to cope with them. We have nine "doors" (*nava dvara*) in our body—two ears, two eyes, two nostrils, a mouth, and two means of elimination—through which we take in the outside world and/or express or eject the inner.

In the Bhakti school, there are nine forms of devotion: hearing (*shravana*) the sacred scriptures, singing (*kirtana*) songs praising the deity, remembering (*smarana*) the divine through meditation, service at the feet of the deity (*pada sevana*), paying homage (*arcana*) to the deity's image, paying obeisance (*vandana*) to the deity, dedicating your actions to the deity as would a servant (*dasya*) or confiding in the deity as would a friend (*sakhya*), and surrendering your Self fully to the deity (*atma nivedana*).[16]

In the *Rama Carita Manasa* (popularly known as the *Ramayana*), the poet Tulsidas lists, through the words of Rama, nine different forms of devotion: always keep to the company of the wise ones; offer humble service at the "lotus feet" of the teacher; sing my praises with a "guileless heart"; repeat my name with "unwavering faith"; practice self-control and virtue; see the world "full of me" without distinction; remain contented with whatever comes your way and never think of detecting others' faults; be "guileless and straight" in dealings with everybody; and in your heart "cherish implicit faith in me without either exultation or depression."[17]

◂ ◂

SEVEN STEPS TO SELF-IGNORANCE
(*AJNANA BHUMIKA*)

When self-knowledge is "disturbed, there arises egotism and bondage.... The delusion that veils ... self-knowledge is sevenfold."
From "The Story of Lavana," in *Vasishtha Yoga*

We're usually instructed by the old texts on the steps we need to take that will reveal to us our true Self. This is typically described as a gradual ascent from the darkness of Self-ignorance to the light of Self-realization, during which the iron grip of the ego is loosened and all the seeming diversity of the world is resolved into Brahman (see chapters 1 and 2), the One. But here we have something a bit unusual: a description of how we devolve from an original condition of pure consciousness to Self-ignorance, in which we're beset by "egotism and bondage."

This descent is fueled by a gradual growth in ego strength and the concomitant feeling of separation from the world around us; in other words, we fall into what monism thinks of as the painful condition of duality (see chapter 1). This downward slide is compared to dropping off into sleep—yet another example of sleep as a metaphor for avidya.

The seven steps are named seed of wakefulness (*bindu jagrat*), wakefulness (*jagrat*), great wakefulness (*maha jagrat*), waking dream (*jagrat svapna*), dream (*svapna*), dreaming wakefulness (*svapna jagrat*), and sleep (*sushupti*).

The seed (*bija*) or substratum of wakefulness of the six succeeding steps is pure consciousness, when "mind (*manas*) and the embodied Self (*jiva*) exist in name only." Here we're reminded that underneath all the turmoil of our surface consciousness, we have access to a state in which there's "no mental agitation, neither distraction nor dullness of mind, neither egotism nor perception of diversity."[18]

Next with wakefulness, we "wake up" with the arousal of a "feeble conception" of the differences between "I" and all that's "not-I." This is the beginning of duality, emphatically condemned by monists (see chapter 1). Remember here that this wakefulness of ours is viewed from a Self-realized yogi's perspective, and so it implies just the opposite of how we typically define the state. Paradoxically, the more wakeful we become in this way, the more deeply we drift off into the sleep of Self-ignorance.

Yoga Sleep (Yoga Nidra)

The yoga tradition is replete with paradoxes that may confuse the untutored beginning student. One of these is the meaning of "yoga sleep" (*yoga nidra*). When the average person is said to be asleep, we all understand they are not only asleep to the world but asleep to themself. But when a yogi is said to be asleep in yoga, they are asleep to the world's duality and awake to their true Self. Yoga sleep then is another phrase for liberation.

◂ ◂

In stage 3, the strengthening of notions of "I" and "not-I" continues apace, fueled by the "memory of previous incarnations." Then our consciousness in stage 4 fully awakens "to its own fancies," holds "undisputed sovereignty over the things of the world," and is filled with and "revels in delight."[19] This leads to a review of all the "false notions" of innumerable experiences passed through as if in a dream, and we remember them as real in the waking state. At the penultimate stage, the dreamer remembers past experiences as if real in the present. Finally in avidyic sleep, past experiences are "abandoned in favor of total inert dullness," and we're "beset with sore pains."[20]

These seven states are "generated out of and perish in the mist of Maya . . . [and] have countless ramifications, each being divided a hundred-fold."[21] After a promising start, we somehow wander off in the wrong direction. Welcome to Self-ignorance.

TWO KINDS OF *DHARMA*: COSMIC AND INDIVIDUAL

In taking the dharma attitude one treats things commonly thought of as other than oneself as oneself . . . in a spirit of respect. . . . The attitude of dharma is an attitude of concern for others as a fundamental extension of oneself.

Karl H. Potter, *Presuppositions of India's Philosophies*

Dharma and karma are usually said to go hand in hand, so to understand the latter, we have to first know something about the former. *Dharma* is one of those Sanskrit words that are difficult if not impossible to translate adequately with just one English word. Essentially though, drawing on its lengthy dictionary definition, *dharma* is the "established order of things," a "steadfast decree," the "law" that "supports" the universe as it evolves and expands.

But *dharma* also means "morality, righteousness, justice, duty." So dharma not only makes sure the world functions smoothly—that the sun rises in the east and sets in the west, that the seasons follow each other in their proper order—but it also regulates the conduct of human society to insure its preservation, progress, and welfare. Though we moderns may be skeptical about and even dismiss such a notion out of hand, traditional India unquestioningly believed that the universe's dharma had a moral dimension that served as the guide and corrective for human behavior.

But this dharma wasn't the same for everyone. It's well-known that Indian society was divided into four basic castes (a simplification of the actual situation, as there were countless subcastes under each of the four): the priests, the rulers and warriors, the merchants and farmers, and the servants. Each of these castes had their own distinct dharma, and it was incumbent on individuals that they adhere to their caste's dharma. If they did so faithfully, then all was well; but if they didn't, if they did something considered *a-dharma*, they were asking for trouble, both from the guardians of the social order and the universe at large.

FOUR KINDS OF ACTIONS (*KARMA*)

Karmma is action, its cause, and effect. There is no uncaused action, nor action without effect. The past, the present, and the future are linked together as one whole.... As the *Brihadaranyaka Upanishad* says: "Man is verily formed of desire. As is his desire, so is his thought. As is his thought, so is his action. As is his action, so is his attainment." These fashion the individual's *karmma*. . . . Then, as to action, "whatsoever a man sows that shall he reap."
Sir John Woodroffe (aka Arthur Avalon), *Mahanirvana Tantra*

How do you view the universe? Is it the product of pure chance, the "fortuitous concourse of atoms," or is it purposeful, the creation of a limitless intelligence with a master plan, however hidden from or beyond our understanding? For most yogis, the workings of the universe have an underlying purpose and harmony, originally called *rita*, which can be translated into something like "divine law." This *rita* is also known as dharma.

For our purposes, we'll define *karma* as "action," though this falls somewhat short of a complete definition. To most people, that word likely suggests only things we actively do or don't do. But as Vyasa interprets Patanjali, action also covers things we say and think, that is, words and thoughts.

There are also two markedly different kinds of action, which we'll call interested and disinterested. The former consists of our typical everyday actions, from which we expect, or at least hope for, a result in our favor—and at the same time hope to avoid one that's not—and which, because of those self-serving expectations, generate more karma. There are three kinds of this karma:[22]

1. Dark (*krishna*) or demeritorious (*adharma*) *karma*, which results from actions that run counter to dharma. There are two kinds of dark karma: (a) external (*bahya*), which is generated in word or deed, and (b) mental (*manasa*), which is generated in thought only.
2. Then there's bright (*shukla*) or meritorious karma, which is mental only. According to Vyasa, it's generated by "those who are engaged in austerities, religious study and meditation," in other words, yogis, the target audience of the *Yoga Sutra*.
3. Finally there's mixed karma, bright and dark (*shukla krishna*), or both meritorious and demeritorious. I guess we can call this gray karma. Gray karma is generated by the average person going about their daily business and is doubtless the most common of the three. (Though we have to wonder, surveying the state of our world—what the yogis see as the Dark Age, the Kali Yuga—if the dark karma is catching up.) This karma is external only, since

all worldly action, despite its surface appearance, is believed to always be an admixture of good and not-so-good.

Disinterested action suggests the opposite of, and is much rarer than, interested. Though technically an action, it's "not-bright not-dark" (*ashukla akrishna*) and usually generated by enlightened beings (*karma sannyasis*) who have renounced the fruit of their actions.

Now as you're probably aware, the consequences of our actions don't always follow on the heels of the actions. Sometimes we'll do something we know is wrong and expect retribution, but then nothing happens and we imagine we pulled the wool over the universe's ever-watchful eyes. Think again, because there are three states of karma:

1. Collected or accumulated (*sancita*) karma is the total stock of karma waiting to be actualized. While waiting, it's gathered in what's called the *karma ashaya*, the "stock of karma," which we carry around with us everywhere we go.
2. Commenced (*prarabdha*) karma, which is being actualized in the current life.
3. Existing (*vartamana*) or "not-going" (*agami*) karma, which is generated in the present life and which will be actualized sometime in the future.

This last state raises an interesting question. What happens to all our existing karma if we die before it's all actualized?

▸ ▸ BEHIND THE NUMBERS

"Born Again and Again" (Punar Janman): *Reincarnation*

In Sanskrit reincarnation is called *punar janman*, literally "go back to birth." What's the story behind this? For the sake of this example, imagine a Self incarnating for the first time. (We'll skip over the question of why an immortal Self wants to put itself through what the yogis perceive as the innate existential suffering of the mundane world.) It lives out its days on Earth in its mortal coil and arrives at the end of its maiden voyage, ready to pass over into the great unknown with much anticipation.

But similar to what many of us have unwisely done with a credit card nowadays, in its life our Self has unavoidably accrued a karmic debt so extensive it can't pay it off in that single incarnation. This extra karma in the store is, as far as I can tell, attached somehow to the subtle body. The universe, like our card's issuing company, is unwilling to forgive the Self its debt, no matter how small, and so it, or at least its accumulated karma carried by its subtle vehicle, is brought back to life to make good on what it owes.

And there's the rub. Our Self reincarnates to work off the karma rolled over from the previous life, but in the process, *it generates more karma*. So at the end of that second life our Self still owes the universe some payback. It returns to embodied life for a third go-round, but at the end of life three, the same situation exists as at the end of life two. This happens again and again and again. If we regard, as the yogis generally do, that to the "discerner (*vivekin*) all is but sorrow,"[23] then it goes without saying our poor Self's situation is unbearable.

The funny part is we have no one to blame for its predicament but ourselves. Our actions in some small way create small blips, like waves on the surface of the ocean, to jiggle the harmonious functioning of the universe, which according to its nature reacts to restore its balance. The universe isn't vindictive; it wants the same thing for us as it wants for itself: Self-realization. Its responses to our actions are neither rewards nor punishments. When it feels an itch, it simply scratches; there's nothing personal involved.

◂ ◂

Now here's where bright karma comes into play. When the Self is reborn, it's not just dropped into life randomly. Three ripenings (*trivipaka*) of its next "wandering through" (*samsara*) are determined by its karma, and it's way better to have more bright in its store than dark. These are:

1. Life-state (*jati*) or the form the Self assumes at birth, which can range from a worm to a human one step away from enlightenment;

in other words, if you have an abundance of bright karma stored up, you can confidently expect to be born into a desirable form. What's the most desirable of all the forms? "Of the 8,400,000 bodily forms, the human body is the most important . . . knowledge of the Essence can't be attained in any other form."[24]

2. Life-time (*ayus*) or the length of time you can anticipate residing in the body before the next great transition.

3. Life-experience (*bhoga*), which depending again on your karmic store, can be either predominantly delightful (*hlada*) or distressing (*paritapa*).

► ► BEHIND THE NUMBERS

Dissenting Voice on Karma and Reincarnation

There's one thing to remember whenever we read something that scholars seem to agree on about the yoga tradition: there will almost always be a dissenting voice or two—reputable scholars who make us wonder if there's anything we can know about the tradition with any certainty. In one way it's maddening, but in another it's something very important that yoga teaches us, and that's to question everything, even the questions.

Most scholars take the connection between karma and reincarnation as gospel, but most isn't everyone. In his *Karma and Creativity*, Christopher Chapple notes that the Hindu monk and Sanskritist Agehananda Bharati (1923–1991) was "quite critical of the karma-reincarnation linkage."[25]

Bharati maintained that modern scholars misunderstood the word *karma*, using it "predominantly in the sense of an impersonal law of positive and negative results due to previous actions." This, in turn, hooked karma up with reincarnation, which wasn't the traditional Indian understanding. Grassroots Hindus never make this connection, he continues, "in most places it means ritualistic action and only that."[26]

◄ ◄

9

MAIN PRACTICES
BY THE NUMBERS

Success is attained by those who practise. How can one attain
success without practise?... Practising alone brings success: this
undoubtedly is the truth.

Svatmarama, *Hatha Yoga Pradipika* 1.65–66

There are two contrasting ways to practice, according to the SU: concentration (*yoga*) and wisdom (*jnana*). The first is to deny—that is, to obstruct the "functioning of the mind" whenever it turns away from the Brahman's existence. This is similar to the process of Classical Yoga, the goal of which is to restrict (*nirodha*) the fluctuations (*vritti*) of consciousness (*citta*) and reveal what's been hidden all the while behind the turmoil, the Self. We might also call this the "path of turning back" (*nivritti marga*—*ni*, "back," *vrt*, "to turn"), away from activity and involvement in the world.

The second way is to affirm, that is, to always remember that in whatever we experience, we have a "clear perception" that there's "nought besides the Brahman." This is similar to the *pratyahara* practice described in the section on the seven withdrawals (see p. 148), in which whatever we see, we're encouraged to look upon "all that as the Atman."[1] This path is *pravritti*, "to turn toward the world" (*pra*, "forth").

Though Shiva is closely identified with the number five, with a few threes tossed in for good measure, he's also known as Ashtamurti, "eight-formed." In one interpretation of this, the eight are the five elements, mind, egotism, and matter (*prakriti*). There's a different eight in the benediction at the start of Kalidasa's play *Shakuntala*:

> Eight forms has Shiva, lord of all and king:
> And these are water, first created thing;
> And fire, which speeds the sacrifice begun;
> The priest; and time's dividers, moon and sun;
> The all-embracing ether, path of sound;
> The earth, wherein all seeds of life are found;
> And air, the breath of life: may he draw near,
> Revealed in these, and bless those gathered here.

The yogis perform a profound obeisance with eight-limb prostration (*ashtanga pranama*), touching to the floor or ground the hands, breast, forehead, eyes, throat, and middle of the back. This phrase can also be applied to a sacrificial offering of eight articles—water, milk, kusha grass, curds, ghee, rice, barley, and mustard—or drop the last three and add honey, red oleander flowers, and sandalwood.

HOW MANY ASANAS ARE THERE?

> There are as many asanas as there are species of creatures. Maheshvara [i.e., Shiva] knows all their varieties. Of the 84 lakhs, one representing each lakh has been cited and thus Shiva has enumerated 84 seats [*pitha*].
>
> *Goraksha Shatakam* 5–6

The old yogis loved large numbers, even into the millions or billions. Such numbers create in us an immediate sense of wonder and awe and remind us how limited our everyday consciousness is when confronted by the immensities of the yoga universe. Of course, such numbers aren't to be taken literally. Like the 40 days and nights of rain Noah endured on his ark, these numbers signify that there's an awful lot of whatever they're counting. Since we humans can't deal easily with extreme numbers, they're typically trimmed down through two or three steps to more human proportions.

One good example of this process starts with the total number of asanas. As we see in the epigraph, Goraksha tells us Shiva, the patron saint of Hatha Yoga, knows as many asanas as there are species of living creatures. How many is that? Eighty-four lakh, according to tradition, and since a lakh equals 100,000, that means there are 8.4 million divinely ordained asanas. Are you impressed? Or overwhelmed?

It's quite obvious that no human has any use for 8.4 million asanas, and so Shiva pared that number down to a way more manageable 84, one one-hundred-thousandth of the original number. There's no indication why these unnamed asanas were singled out, except that Shiva somehow determined they're preeminent (*visishta*).[2]

The GS stops with the 32 "most useful" asanas, though it's not explained how or why they're so. The 32 are listed at GS 2.3–6, leaving us to wonder both about the names of the less useful 52 and, more relevant to our subject, if the number 32 has any significance (which we'll look at in this chapter).

Svatmarama in the HYP takes the paring one step farther, or maybe one step lower. He completes his asana chapter with the four he believes are the most excellent (*sarabhuta*) of all. Imagine. Start out with 8.4 million asanas, now just four are left, and once again, we have this number standing for something complete and excellent. In a way, this very small number is somehow just as remarkable as its source: all those millions and millions of asanas whittled down to these special few. So what are they? You might pause for a moment and speculate on what you think they are; there may be a surprise or two in what comes next.

We first should acknowledge that the Fab Four are all sitting poses—maybe one of those surprises I just mentioned. Most modern students, when asked to guess which poses are "most excellent," reveal their modern bias for active poses. We don't usually realize how central pranayama and meditation—performed while sitting—were to the traditional practice.

The best-known member of the four is one of the most iconic poses, Lotus (*padmasana*).[3] There's no question why it's included. According to Svatmarama, it destroys sickness, bestows "unparalleled knowledge" from the power of the goddess, and sitting in this pose with breath restrained guarantees liberation "without a doubt" (*natra samshaya*), which seems overly optimistic.[4]

The next two poses are each a surprise in their own way. First we have Blessed Pose (*bhadrasana*),[5] what today we call Bound Angle (*baddha konasana*). Blessed is something of a letdown after Lotus, as all it does is destroy disease. That's not a minor benefit surely, but nothing like its flowery companion's promise.

Then there's Lion Pose (*simhasana*),[6] the one pose among the four that nobody ever guesses. Why this one? Svatmarama calls it "most elevated" (*uttama*) because it joins the three *bandhas*, the bonds at the throat (*jalandhara*), perineum (*mula*), and abdomen (*uddiyana*) essential for pranayama. Here with the inclusion of Lion, we see another example of the importance of formal breathing in the tradition. By the way, there's no mention in the text of the roaring sound that we create in the pose's modern version.

Finally the pose Svatmarama deems the best (*mukhya*) of all the asanas is Adept Pose (*siddhasana*). Fittingly, he devotes nine verses to this pose, more than any of the other 14 poses he includes in the text, even Lotus, which "only" rates six verses. Adept purifies the nadis (important as a prep for pranayama) and, like Lion, encourages the three bandhas, but most of all (along with meditating on the Self and eating a moderate diet), the pose with regular practice after just 12 years, "opens the door to liberation."[7]

▸ ▸ BEHIND THE NUMBERS

How Many Asanas Are There in Modern Yoga?

While we modern yogis come up a bit short of 8.4 million asanas, we still have a pretty fair number to keep us occupied. I have a copy of the *Encyclopaedia of Traditional Asanas,* compiled by the Lonavla Yoga

Institute of Lonavla, India, published in 2006. The editors surveyed 160 texts and manuscripts, both ancient and modern (but not Iyengar's *Light on Yoga*), and according to the book's dust cover, came up with "approximately 900 titles of asanas." We also have *Light on Yoga*, which includes 198 asanas (and two mudras). It's safe to say then that we have access to at least a thousand asanas, likely more.

▸ ▸ BEHIND THE NUMBERS

84 in Sanskrit

Eighty-four in Sanskrit is *caturashiti*.

We might ask: what's the significance of 84, if any? According to S. Dasgupta, "it has been rightly held by some scholars that this number eighty-four is rather a mystic than a historical number."[8] For examples, he notes that the Ajivikas believe the soul must pass through 840,000 stages before becoming human, that the MaiU[9] and some Puranas mention the same number of states of birth, and that the Kanphata yogis sometimes have rosaries (*mala*) with 84 beads instead of the customary 108. Gudrun Bühnemann, in her comprehensive review of *Eighty-four Asanas in Yoga*, notes that the number "signifies completeness, and in some cases, sacredness."[10]

Some writers try to explain the import of 84 by pointing out that it's a product of other recognizably symbolic or sacred numbers. Seven times 12 is quite popular. For John Campbell Oman in *The Mystics, Ascetics, and Saints of India* (1905), seven represents the number of so-called "classical planets" in Indian astrology (the Sun and Moon, Mercury, Venus, Mars, Jupiter and Saturn), and 12, the number of signs in the zodiac. What the asanas have to do with astrology though, isn't explained. Matthew Kapstein gives seven and 12 a slightly different spin, noting that from a "numerological point of view," both are related to three and four, the former as the sum of the two numbers ($3 + 4 = 7$), the latter as the product ($3 \times 4 = 12$). By then multiplying the sum by the product, we arrive at our 84. Kapstein remarks that symbolically 84 "encompasses the range of possible relationships obtaining among the innumerable magical and natural categories involving threes and fours," though unfortunately he doesn't provide any specific examples. However from a "historical perspective," he concludes, 84 is "entirely arbitrary."[11]

▸ ▸ BEHIND THE NUMBERS

32 in Sanskrit

Thirty-two in Sanskrit is *dvatrimshat*.

Symbolically, 32 isn't your typical meaning-laden number, like, say, nine or 12, nor does it seem to be significantly related in any way to any other number of recognized significance, like 72, 84, or 108. I did turn up one curious parallel though. In the first chapter of the HYP, we have Svatmarama's roster of the 32 great adepts (*maha siddhas*).[12] This is a lineage of yogis—beginning with the "first lord," Shiva—who've "broken Time's staff" (*kala danda*, an emblem of the god of death, Yama) and freely wander about in Brahma's egg (*brahma anda*, see p. 33); in other words, they've conquered both time (and so death) and space. Does the 32 in Svatmarama have an echo in the 32 of Gheranda? The latter certainly was familiar with the former, since descriptions of half-dozen asanas in the GS are the same or very close to those in the earlier text (e.g., compare HYP 1.32 with GS 2.19). Could the choice of 32 asanas be a subtle tribute to the 32 adepts? This is probably just wishful thinking on my part, and anyway, and even if true, it just switches the question about the number to a different text.

◂ ◂

TWO KINDS OF SEALS (*MUDRA*): HAND (*HASTA*) AND BODY (*KAYA*)

Mudras are formed with great care; they are prescribed with great discrimination. Behind the science of the Mudras ages of practice alone stand as proof.

B. Bhattacharya, *Shaivism and the Phallic World*

Mudras can be classified in four or five different ways; we'll look at three here. The mudras most familiar to most students are the hand mudras (*hasta mudra*). Like many practices the yogis engage in, these mudras have both a symbolic meaning and a practical use. Symbolically, mudras are "archetypal signs, based on gestural finger patterns." They're used to "evoke in the mind ideas symbolizing divine powers or deities themselves in order to intensify the adept's concentration."[13] Mudras are also used to quiet the fingers and hands, since any small movements of the body will disturb the meditating brain.

Just as we can't say for sure how many types of gurus and initiations there are, it's also not possible to get a firm number on mudras. John Woodroffe, in his introduction to the MNT, numbers them at 108, but this is primarily a symbolic number. Cain and Revital Carroll, in their excellent *Mudras of India: A Comprehensive Guide to the Hand Gestures of Yoga and Indian Dance* (2012), collected by my rough count 103 yoga mudras (and a large number of gestures used in Indian dance which I didn't count).

According to the Carrolls, hand seals are used to "regulate the flow of *prana* . . . and ready the mind for meditation."[14] Woodroffe notes that mudras are used for worship, chanting, and bathing, among other things.[15]

Georg Feuerstein once told me it was possible the hand seals originated with Vedic students. Benjamin Walker similarly speculates they might be traced to the "positions taken by the hand in the mnemotechnical finger-devices called *samahasta*, used by Vedic reciters to remember the accent and stress of the sacred chant."[16]

▸ ▸ BEHIND THE NUMBERS

Two Meanings of Mudra

A very long time ago, envelopes were sealed with a dollop of hot wax pressed by a special ring, called a signet ring. The ring left a particular impression in the wax, indicating to those in the know who had sealed the envelope. The yogis would call this ring a mudra. Literally when applied to the human body, a mudra is a "seal" with a double meaning. In one sense, the mudra seals something in the body, typically vital energy or prana. In another sense, just as the ring seals the identity of the person in the wax, a mudra seals the identity of the deity associated on the practitioner.

The figurative definition indicates that a mudra is so-named because it pleases (*mudam*) the gods and "melts the mind" (*drava*).[17] Incidentally, mudra is another one of those Sanskrit words that are usually mispronounced by us English speakers. We typically emphasize the first syllable, MOO-druh. That's actually a word meaning "joyous, glad." But the mudra we're talking about here is spelled with a long final *a*, which gets the emphasis and so is pronounced, moo-DRAH.

▸ ▸ PRACTICE

Jnana Mudra (Wisdom Seal)

Jnana mudra might be the most widely known of the hand seals. It's quite easy to perform. Simply touch the tips of your index fingers and thumbs, creating a circle, and gently curl the other three fingers away. The way it's been explained to me is that the index finger represents the embodied Self (*jivatman*), the thumb the supreme Self (*paramatman* or Brahman), and touching them stands for union (*yoga*). The remaining fingers are the three strands (*guna*) of matter: tamas, rajas, and sattva. Laying your hands palms down on your knees creates jnana mudra or the wisdom seal; palms up creates cin mudra, the "consciousness seal."

According to the Carrolls, jnana "sharpens the intellect . . . during meditation, lifts depression," and "opens the lower lobes of the lungs."[18] Cin mudra has much the same effect. "It calms the mind, opens the chest for breathing, and 'seals' energy in the body to increase the benefits of any asana."[19] (Just to be clear, I haven't been able to confirm any of these benefits, but that's just me).

◂ ◂

The second type of mudra is the body (*kaya*) mudra. Judging by our Western yoga in the twenty-first century, we might imagine that asana has always been central to Hatha Yoga. But we'd be mistaken. The central technique of early HY is this body seal, with its subset of bonds or bandhas. Svatmarama included 10 mudras in the HYP, taking up most of the third chapter. Gheranda ups the ante in the third chapter of the GS to 25. Body mudras come in all shapes and sizes. They make use of (in no particular order) the tongue, eyes, belly, anal sphincter, and several of them would be or are today considered as asanas. The most prevalent of this latter group was once known as *viparita karani mudra*, the "inverted making seal," but nowadays is commonly called Shoulder Stand (*sarvangasana*).

Any number of physical benefits are claimed for this pose, which may or may not have any factual bases. Originally though, viparita karani had one very specific purpose, and that was to prevent the precious elixir of immortality (*amrita* or *soma*) from dripping down from its source in the head and being burned up and so wasted in the solar plexus.

▸ ▸ BEHIND THE NUMBERS

Amrita: The Elixir of Immortality

> The Sun (at the navel) draws (to himself) the stream of nectar flowing from the Moon (at the base of the palate). . . . The navel is up and the palate is below. . . . This action [is] known as Viparita Karani.
>
> *Goraksha Shatakam* 54, 59

In each of us, says the tradition, there's a subtle organ at the back of our throat—or maybe the base of our brain—that secretes a subtle elixir that, if properly preserved and sipped, would extend our lives far past the normal span of years. But whenever we're in the upright position, which is likely a good part of the day, the precious elixir drip, drip, drips down from the back of our throat into our belly, where it's incinerated, its promise tragically wasted in the fiery solar plexus.

The yogis have known about a very simple way to preserve this elixir for probably something like 600 years, maybe more. The solution is staring us right in the, um, feet. If the elixir drips down as long as our head is above our belly, the obvious solution is to raise our belly above our head. Seem familiar? That would end the leakage, and the elixir would be withdrawn and stored in our head for easy access. Originally this position was called the "reverse action seal" (*viparita karani mudra*), but is nowadays known as Shoulder Stand (*sarvangasana*). This practice is also considered a "withdrawal," or pratyahara (see p. 148).

Shoulder Stand is one of the traditional poses that have been repurposed for modern times. The section in Iyengar's *Light on Yoga* recounting the effects of this pose is one of the longest of its kind in the book. Shoulder Stand is promoted as the cure for everything from a common cold to epilepsy. With all due respect, I would read this section with a modicum of skepticism.

◄ ◄

THREE BONDS (*BANDHA*)

Traditionally, bandhas were classified as part of mudras. . . . The *Hatha Yoga Pradipika* deals with bandhas and mudras together and the ancient tantric texts also make no distinction between the two.

Swami Satyananda Saraswati,
Asana Pranayama Mudra Bandha

The three bandhas apply especially to the practice of pranayama, in particular when the goal of the practice is the awakening of the dormant spiritual energy (Kundalini) ensconced at the base of the spine in the root cakra. The torso in this process is visualized as a pot (*kumbha*, *ghata*); in fact, Gheranda calls his teaching the "yoga of the pot."[20] We can think of this pot as something akin to a pressure cooker, which heats the vital energy retained in the torso, which in turn is used to stimulate the Kundalini into action.

But first the pot—which has two openings at the anus and throat—must be sealed tight so no energy can leak out. This is done with the root bond (*mula bandha*), in which the base of the pelvis and anal sphincter are contracted to close off the bottom opening, and the throat bond (*kantha bandha*)—usually called *jalandhara bandha*, the "net holding bond" (*jala*, "net," *adhara*, "hold")—in which the top of the sternum is joined to the chin to close off the throat. This then contains the prana securely in the torso during breath retention (*kumbhaka*, "pot-like").

But that's not all. In order to heat the prana, the apana vayu resident in the pelvis and the prana vayu resident in the chest must be joined with the samana vayu in the abdomen (see p. 67). To do this, the natural tendency of apana to descend and prana to ascend must be reversed. This is the second job of the mula and kantha bandhas: the former lifts apana; the latter pushes down prana. Once the three vayus are joined in the lower abdomen, *uddiyana bandha*, the "flying up bond," is applied. This is accomplished by an extreme contraction of the abdominal muscle (rectus abdominis), drawing it back toward the spine and so compressing the retained prana. Like the contents of a pressure cooker, the prana is heated to its metaphorical boiling point, which then rouses the Kundalini.

EIGHT TRADITIONAL BREATHS (*PRANAYAMA*)

Eight: A symbol of entrance into a new state or condition of the soul, the number seven signifying completion of the former state.

G. A. Gaskell, *Dictionary of All Scriptures and Myths*

These are the eight kumbhakas: *surya bhedana, ujjayi, sitkari, shitali, bhastrika, bhramari, murccha,* and *plavini.*

Hatha Yoga Pradipika 2.44

The most common number for included breaths in the old Hatha texts is eight, in which there's a faint echo, intentional or not, of Patanjali's eight limbs. The breaths in the HYP set the stage for later texts. Six of its eight—Sun Piercing (*surya bhedana*), Conqueror (*ujjayi*), Seet Making (*sitkari*), Cooling (*shitali*), Bellows (*bhastrika*), and Bee (*bhramari*)—

with one or two exceptions, are generally instructed in subsequent texts—at least the ones I have access to. These six are also current today: all are found in B.K.S. Iyengar's influential *Light on Pranayama*.

The remaining two—Swooning (*murccha*) and Floater (*plavini*)—have, as far as I can tell, fallen out of favor. The former seems to involve a long retention after inhalation, followed by a slow exhale that "clears the mind and brings happiness."[21] The latter asks us to fill the belly with air—it can be done—and "float happily like a lotus leaf" in water.[22] It's not clear from the text if we should do this as part of the practice or that we could do it if we've a mind to. The Bihar School of Yoga's commentary on the verse says that Floater is useful in cases of gastritis and stomach acidity and to fill the stomach to ward off hunger pangs when fasting. This pair is usually not found in subsequent texts.

Following these eight, the HYP treats Connected (*sahita*) and Unconnected (*kevala*) retentions or breath holding (*kumbhaka*). The former seems to be the preliminary stage for the latter, though neither is described in much detail. There's a rather cryptic comment that kevala is freedom from inhalation and exhalation.[23] This appears to be, if I'm not mistaken, what Patanjali called the "Fourth" (*caturtha*) breath,[24] that transcends inhale and exhale.

About 250 years later, these two retentions show up as members of the eight breaths in the GS, which drops Seet Making and Floater. Here Connected seems to be what we today know as alternate nostril breathing, which has two kinds, seeded—that is, with a mantra (OM)—and unseeded, without. Unconnected is the spontaneous confinement of the breath in the body. Yogi Pranavananda deems it the "crown of pranayama. It is a point where movement and rest co-exist in perfect equilibrium."[25] In a note to HRA 2.28, the editors of the text explain that kevali is an "advanced stage of *sahita* . . . and is attained irrespective of inhalation or exhalation. Thus sahita . . . is voluntary, whereas *kevala* is involuntary."[26]

Most of the other texts I looked through included the six breaths still around today and typically either or both Connected and Unconnected. The *Hatha Tatva Kaumudi*, a monumental work of 56 chapters and 720 pages in my translation, includes all eight breaths from the HYP and then adds another 14 breaths, with names like Drawing Down (*apakar-sha*) and Moving the Jiva (*jivacala*). Practices include various manipulations of the nostrils, retentions, and breathing meditations on the cakras.

SEVEN WITHDRAWALS (*PRATYAHARA*)

> As a turtle, after having seen a danger, contracts all the parts of the body in a moment, in the same way a wise person should withdraw his or her senses from their objects.
>
> *Brihad Yogi Yajnavalkya Smriti* 8.51–52

A common definition of *pratyahara* is the "withdrawal of the senses from their objects." This is Patanjali's version of the practice, the fifth of his eight limbs.[27] Because of the widespread popularity of the YS among students in the West, we tend to assume that Patanjali's practice is definitive, but this isn't quite right. We know, for example, that scattered throughout traditional literature are far more yamas and niyamas than the five of each listed by Patanjali. The same is true for pratyahara, which is used to name at least six other practices—and there may be a few more that I missed—that have nothing to do with sense withdrawal.

Plainly opposed to Patanjali's version is a pratyahara that urges us to look upon all we see "as the Atman."[28] Seeing the Atman "in the objects of desire" creates, according to the TBU, a "pleasant experience of the mind."[29] Rather than retreat from the world into a self-contained cocoon, this practice invites us to dive into the world headfirst and envision the Self in all we see as the same Self that animates and supports our own lives. With this, all sense of separation between our truest Self and those of others is eradicated. What I like about the approach of the TBU is that its objects of desire aren't dismissed out of hand, but instead we're prompted to enjoy them as they should be by finding the Self residing in them. This same approach is echoed in the Tamil language *Tiru Mantiram*, a poem of about 3,000 verses by the sage Tirumular.

> In the act of pratyahara
> All the world will be visioned;

Be rid of the despicable darkness
And seek the Lord;
If your thoughts be centered firm
You shall divine light see
And immortal thereafter be.[30]

The next pratyahara shifts the emphasis from seeing to doing. "Whatever one does, whether pure or impure, till the moment of his death, all that, he should do unto the Brahman."[31] This is, as I understand it, a form of Karma Yoga, in which all our actions, even though they're "impure," are humbly and unstintingly dedicated to the Absolute. By conducting ourselves in this way, with the beneficiary of our life's work always in the back of our mind, we'll be conscious of making each of our offerings worthy of its recipient.

The fourth pratyahara is probably best considered as a subset of the second. Apparently this one was originally directed to the Hindu house-holder (*grihastha*), whose life was considerably more ritualized than ours is today. The practice is to perform "daily ceremonial observances" with the "mental attitude" that they're meant to gain the goodwill of the Absolute.[32] No doubt we lack the many formal ceremonies incumbent on a Hindu householder. Nevertheless, to practice this kind of pratyahara, we might transform our more common and frequent household chores that because of their familiarity often slip through the cracks of our awareness into simple rituals that even the Absolute would be pleased to accept.

The fifth pratyahara, as I understand it, is a meditation on the identity of, or nondifference between, our embodied Self (*jivatman*) and the supreme Self (*paramatman*), the Absolute. Here we're instructed to "mentally abstract" the idea of the atman in our body, and then "confine" that abstraction in the "non-dual, indeterminate" Absolute. If we practice this, says the text, "nothing is unattainable."[33]

The breathing practice that makes up the sixth pratyahara requires a vivid imagination. Here we're directed to breathe into a predetermined sequence of body parts or organs, sometimes 18 in number, other times

16. At each station in the sequence, we retain the breath there for a limited time, say three to five seconds, then withdraw it and, "peacefully" as one text puts it, proceed to the next station in the sequence, repeating the retention and withdrawal at each station until the sequence comes to its end, typically at the crown. Then we reverse the sequence and return to the big toes. You can sit or recline for this practice.

▸ ▸ PRACTICE

Withdrawal Breathing with the 18 Props (Adhara)

I found about a half-dozen sequences of what we'll call breathing pratyahara in different texts. I thought you might like to try this exercise, so here's a list of the 12 most commonly named parts or organs, followed by a list of parts or organs that showed up in only one sequence. I decided to omit the organs of reproduction and elimination. Usually the awareness proceeds up through the body, stopping to breathe in each of the adharas you've chosen for your sequence. When you reach your crown, reverse the sequence and return finally to your toes.

Possible adharas: big toes, ankles, midcalves, knees, midthighs, groins, navel, heart, throat, midbrow between the eyebrows, forehead, crown. Extras: heels, elbows, hands, tongue.

▸ ▸ BEHIND THE NUMBERS

The 18 Family and 108

Eighteen in Sanskrit is *ashtadashan*, 108 is *ashtottarashata*, literally, "eight more than a hundred (*shata*)."

There are certain things in our modern world that are immediately associated with traditional yoga, often by people not even part of the yoga community. The lotus (*padma*) would be one, along with someone sitting in the asana of the same name, *padmasana*. The OM sigil would be another, and the figure of Shiva Nataraja, the "lord of the dance."

Then there's the number 108. Have you ever been challenged in a class—as I have several times over the years—to perform 108 Sun Salutes?

Have you ever taken a workshop for which the fee was $108? Do you own a mala? There's a good chance it's strung with 108 beads. We've all been led to believe 108 is somehow special, even sacred, though we might be hard pressed to explain exactly why. Theories proposing the meaning and origin of 108 abound, but so far none has managed to gain wide acceptance.

Actually, 108 is the most visible member of what we can call the 18 family—the members of which are 18 and its multiples and variants (e.g., $18 \times 4 = 72$; $18 \times 6 = 108$; $108 \times 3 = 216$; $216 + 216 = 432$). Eighteen itself has a prominent place in India's most beloved tale, the sprawling epic poem the *Mahabharata*, reputedly the longest poem in existence. It's divided into 18 chapters, the combatants in the climactic civil war are divided into 18 armies—11 on one side, seven on the other—and the bloody battle itself raged on for 18 days. The revered spiritual poem extracted from this epic, the *Bhagavad Gita*, also has 18 chapters. There are a few more 18s associated with the epic, but research suggests they're more wishful thinking than actual facts.

We might also note that 18 times 4 equals 72, and if we tack on three zeros, we'll have the number of nadis in the subtle body, 72,000. In Indian Ayurvedic medicine, the subtle body is also peppered with 107 energy joints (*marman*), reminiscent of acupuncture points, with the skin linking all the joints together considered as the 108th marman.

But the MaB and the BG aren't the only significant bearers of 18. The venerated text at the heart of orthodox Hindu spirituality, the RV, is said to be composed in what's called *pankti* meter (*pankti*, "collection of five," though the text is actually written in verses of various numbers of syllables). *Pankti* is a stanza consisting of five lines of eight syllables each, for a total of 40 syllables. It's further claimed there are 10,800 verses in the text, and since each of these verses has 40 syllables, the RV supposedly has $10,800 \times 40$ or 432,000 syllables total. We also know that Vedic priests conducted a sacrifice at an altar, usually shaped like a bird, constructed of 10,800 kiln-fired bricks, each one put in place very precisely and accompanied with a mantra.

The books that comprise the concluding portion of the Vedic canon, collectively known as the Upanishads, are traditionally numbered at 108, though scholars estimate there are anywhere from 150 to over 200 of these texts. "If you long after 'bodiless liberation' (*videha mukti*)," advises the seventeenth-century *Muktipa Upanishad*, "study the 108 Upanishads,"[34] which it then goes on to list. Then too, there 18 *maha* or major Puranas, the sacred tales of ancient times, along with 18 secondary (*upa*) Puranas, though like the 108 Upanishads, there are many more than 18 of these texts.

The yogis estimate we take 15 breaths each minute, which is fairly accurate for resting adults. (Children breathe much faster.) This works out to 900 breaths each hour, 10,800 each half day, and 21,600 in one day.

We're also informed that one of the best times of the day to practice breathing and meditation is just before sunrise. This is called the hour of Brahma (*brahma muhurta*). There was a time in India when each day was measured out in 30 *muhurtas* ("moments"), which lasted 48 minutes each. If we multiply 360, the symbolical number of days in a year, by the number of muhurtas in a day, 30, we'll find there are 10,800 muhurtas in a year.

Speaking of years, recall from chapter 3 that our current age, the Kali Yuga, is scheduled to last 432,000 years, a maha yuga totals 10 times that number, 4,320,000 years, and one day in the life of Brahma, called a kalpa, equals 2,000 *maha yugas*, or 8,640,000,000 years.

Finally, maybe the most well-known use of 108 applies to the number of beads on a mala or rosary, designed to help a reciter of mantras (*japaka*) keep track of their recitations. The number of beads, the material from which the beads are made, the times of day suitable for the practice, the best place for the practice, the material of the seat on which the japaka sits, the pose in which the japaka sits and the direction faced, these aspects and more are all strictly governed by tradition.

Now we might think that 108 is the standard number of beads strung on a mala. But over the centuries we find references to malas with beads ranging generally from the midteens to the mid-80s, though some even exceed 108. For example, in Yogaraja's commentary on Abhinavagupta's tenth-century CE text titled *Paramarthasara*, he makes reference to a mala with 244 beads.[35] Some of these numbers are relatable to 108, such as 18 and 27 (108 ÷ 4), while others have no intrinsic relationship at all (e.g., 15, 30, 50). Remember then that though 108 beads are very common for a mala, it's not the only number possible.

> It [i.e., a mala] is hung around the neck [of the yogi] and consists of thirty-two, or sixty-four, or one hundred and eight, or even of more berries. A smaller one having eighteen or twenty-eight berries, is worn on the wrist or elbow.[36]

Such examples could be continued on and on, not only selected from Hinduism and Indian culture, but from other religions and ancient cultures all over the world. But all of this raises a pressing question, which is: why? Why is 108 so revered and ubiquitous? The short answer is, as I've already noted, nobody knows for sure, or we could say, there are people who believe they know for sure, but none have been able to garner widespread agreement. Here are three of the most common reasons given.

One hundred eight is the result of the multiplication of two sacred numbers in their own right, typically nine and 12. The reasoning goes that if we multiply these two numbers together, the result of 108 must also be sacred. This naturally leads to the question: why are nine and 12 considered sacred?

Cultural historian Fredrick Bunce declares nine to be a "perfect number," a "magnification" of the sacred number three, and "by association and as a derivation of from three" ($3 + 3 + 3 = 9$; $3 \times 3 = 9$; $\sqrt{9} = 3$), "nine also becomes one of the most sacred numbers." It denotes "completion, perfection, force, wisdom, silence."[37] Bunce then finds 12 to be an "auspicious cosmic number" that denotes "sacrifice and is related to immortality."[38] We might question why it's only the multiplication of these two numbers that results in a sacred number. What about addition? Why isn't 21 considered equally sacred?

A second possible solution is what we can call the astrology justification, which involves nine and 12 again or four and 27. Vedic astrology has nine planets (*graha*) and 12 houses (*bhava*) in its system, which is considered sacred. Belonging then to what's considered a sacred system, the result of nine times 12 is similarly sacred. A second astrological approach to 108 multiplies the 27 lunar mansions (*nakshatra*), thought of as dwellings for the gods, times their four quarters (*pada*).

I should point out that just five of the Vedic astrologer's nine planets—Mercury, Venus, Mars, Jupiter, and Saturn—are what we think of as planets in the West. The other four are the sun and our moon, a star and satellite, and a pair of lunar nodes, the Northern (*rahu*) and Southern (*ketu*), which aren't physical bodies, but rather two imaginary points in space where the paths of the sun and moon intersect as they move around the celestial sphere.

Speaking of the sun and moon, a third rather ingenious reason given for 108's special status is based, believe it or not, on calculations using the diameters of Earth (7,917 miles), sun (864,337 miles), and moon (2,159 miles), and the distances between them (Earth to sun: 92,955,807 miles; Earth to moon: 238,900 miles). There are three versions.

The first calculation involves the distance from Earth to the sun, which is supposed to be 108 times the diameter of the sun. So we have: 92,955,807 ÷ 864,337 = 107.5, not a bad approximation. The second calculation involves the distance from Earth to the moon, which is supposed to be 108 times the moon's diameter. So we have: 238,900 ÷ 2,158 = 110.7, again, not bad. Finally, the third calculation says we'll derive 108 if we divide the sun's diameter by that of the Earth. So we have: 865,370 ÷ 7,917 = 109.3.

The question here is: were the ancient Indian astronomers savvy enough to figure out these distances and diameters using what are by modern standards rather unsophisticated methods? Apparently, while it's not entirely impossible they could have, we can't really tell how close they came owing to the difference of their standards of measurement."[39]

◀ ◀

10

MANTRA BY THE NUMBERS

The entire universe is of the nature of consciousness, which is nothing but reflection nature, and that again is, in essence, sound.

H.N. Chakravarty, trans., *Tantrasara of Abhinavagupta*

The world is filled with sound. Some sound is natural, like thunder or the wind shushing through the trees. Some sound is human made, like strumming a guitar or a plane passing overhead. Some sound is made by living creatures, like chirping birds or human voices. Some sound is even "inaudible"—though only so to creatures, like us, whose hearing range extends from 20 to 20,000 hertz. There are plenty of creatures that can hear sounds below or above that range, and with the right instruments, we can hear them too, albeit secondhand. One thing all these sounds have in common though is that they're what the yogis call "struck" (*ahata*), they have a detectable source, such as two solid things hitting together or air vibrating a vocal apparatus. All of this is the concern of the science of sound: acoustics.

It shouldn't come as a surprise that the yogis have their own science of sound, but as usual with them, it begins and ends with the Self. They locate the source of all sound in what they call *shabda Brahman*, Absolute sound. Since *shabda* is pure consciousness, its sound, in contrast to our everyday struck sound, is said to be "unstruck" (*anahata*). What exactly does that mean, *unstruck sound*?

Extensive research into this question found general phrases like "mystical sound" and the "sound of the celestial realm," neither of which is especially informative. The most substantial definition I found of what is called shabda is "consciousness itself where thought and word are the same and not yet distinguished. Brahman is the eternal word from which emanates everything."[1] Obviously the concept of a sound that's unstruck is completely alien to anything we've ever experienced, and though shabda itself is the source of words, words can't pin it down, much as we saw with nirguna Brahman.

Whatever it is, we can't hear unstruck sound with our ears, not even if we're hooked up to the most sensitive sound-detecting instrument. In order to express itself then, shabda must pass through three stages, which is compared to a plant growing from a seed.

The second phase, which "sprouts" from shabda Brahman, is literally called "visible sound" (*pashyanti shabda*). At first glance this seems like an odd name for sound, until we see in the dictionary it also means "rightly understanding." While "thought and word" are still not distinguished, pashyanti is a kind of desire, or maybe more of a wish, to "rightly understand" all the countless possible ways it could express itself. The YSU says of this stage that the "means of which the Yogis see the universe, they know it as Pashyanti."[2]

From pashyanti buds the third stage, called "middle sound" (*madhyama shabda*), sandwiched as it is between the second and fourth stages, between the sheer potential of sound and that sound's manifestation. Middle sound is also known as "hidden speech" because it's associated with ideation and reason. With this stage we're finally in familiar territory, where the inchoate desire of pashyanti is transformed into a concrete idea, and words are right on the tip of our tongue. The YSU locates madhyama in the heart, where it "resembles that of a thundering cloud" we can assume ready to pour out its words through our lips.[3]

Finally madhyama blossoms into corporeal or tangible speech (*vaikhari shabda*), but now we have a much different attitude toward our words. Since the source is shabda, each of our words is invested, as the YSU reports, "by the grace of the Goddess of Learning," Sarasvati, with a "remarkable power." The text assures us that whoever wields such power will, of their own accord, become the "author of Vedas, Shastras and Puranas," in other words, words of sublime wisdom.[4]

We all believe that our words are struck—the result of "two solid things hitting together or air vibrating a vocal apparatus," nothing but acoustics. But the yogis tell us otherwise, that our words have their ultimate source in the unstruck Absolute. Every word we speak has a divine origin, much like a mantra, and a depth of meaning of which we're hardly, if at all, aware.

But there's something else about this process that's of even greater importance to the yogis, which is that it can be reversed. The yogis start with vaikhari as if on the bottom rung of a ladder, and climb back through madhyama and pashyanti to return to the source and Self-realization.

Speech which had its origin in the above-said manner, will, when the order is reversed, reach the vanishing stage. Of that organ of speech, the supreme lord is the eternal and immutable Paramatman, who rouses the power of speech. That person who always rests in the conviction "I am it," is in no way affected, even though spoken to in articulate sounds, high, low or vulgar.[5]

TWO FORMS OF RECITATION (*JAPA*)

Japa is an auspicious giver of enjoyment, salvation, and self-fulfilling wish.

Kularnava Tantra 15.5

We've come to expect in traditional yoga that very few practices are simple and straightforward. The old yogis seem to revel in making things as difficult as possible for themselves. This was likely done first to weed out the dilettantes from the true believers and then to put the latter through the mill to grind down their egos until there was nothing left. This would presumably open their consciousness to higher dimensions, although we have to assume, I believe, that the process didn't always work out as planned.

The YY defines *japa* as "repeating in the proper manner" a mantra received from the guru.[6] There are two things to note here. Mantras recited improperly have no transformative power. In the proper manner, due attention is paid to the mantra's meter—if it's more than one syllable—and its meaning; in other words, we shouldn't do our japa with an "uncontrolled mind."[7] Also, traditionally, mantras must be given to us by a Self-realized teacher, who can peer into our Self and understand just what we need to further our spiritual maturation. Mantras drawn from a book are frowned upon. In a few of the old texts, japa is included among 10 niyamas.[8] The HRA has two sets of niyamas, 10 for the mind and 10 for the body, and japa is included in the latter category.[9]

Now there are several preliminary dos and don'ts for japa according to tradition, which apply mostly to ascetics. The specific place and the surrounding area where the yogi does japa are important. At the low end of place for benefit is a house, and then in ascending order they are near a river, in a cow pen, in a place with a sacred fire, at a place of pilgrimage, and finally near a deity like Vishnu or Shiva, where the benefit is infinite. As with yoga in general, the ascetic's country should be peaceful and well-governed, which in this day and age is likely harder to find than a cow pen. There's a whole lot more regarding the traditional practice of japa, even recommendations on what foods to eat (including something called *caru*, rice boiled in butter and milk), but I think it's clear from what I've just covered that the yogis consider it serious business.

Now about the actual practice itself. According to the *Brihad Yogi Yajnavalkya Smriti* (BYY) and several other texts, there are two general ways to perform japa.[10] The first is called "consisting of words" (*vacika*), which in turn consists of two types. The first of these is familiar to most of us, that is, reciting the mantra out loud. This is called "noisy" (*sashabda*) or "loud" (*uccais*) japa, which is thought to be exercising. The second kind of vacika is called *upamshu* or "whispered" japa, which lowers the volume to a minimum and is said to be nourishing, as whispering always is. Whispered japa is 1,000 times better than spoken. It's suggested that the deity being addressed by the mantra must perforce come closer to the chanter to better hear what's being chanted in its honor or suppliance, or that it's just to foil any prying ears from receiving a vicarious benefit from our practice.

The second general way to perform japa is called "mental" (*manasa*) japa, which as the name implies is done without speaking aloud. The DU further subdivides mental japa into two types, one in which we "reflect" (*manana*) on the mantra in our mind only, the other done while in meditation (*dhyana*).[11] In either case, mental japa is said to be tranquilizing, as we might expect from a word or words intensely repeated over time.

The practice should ideally be done away from other people in secrecy. Otherwise, if someone overhears us, all the benefits are lost. When doing manasa japa, we're instructed not to move our tongue or lips, shake our head and neck, or show our teeth. This is supposed to prevent "ghosts, demons and spirits, semi-divine beings, supernatural beings and semi-divine serpents" from reading our lips to discover our mantra and then forcibly seizing the hard-earned fruits of our labor for themselves.[12] Just as whispered japa exceeds spoken japa, the benefits of silent mantra far exceed those of both the spoken versions. This might come as a surprise, as accustomed as we are to repeating mantras with a full-throated, rousing sound. It's said that the benefit of manana japa is 1,000 times greater than whispered, while dhyana japa beats out manana by another 1,000 times. Be aware, though, that the SSP apparently contradicts all this, instructing us to do our *japa* "without any expectations."[13]

So why is silent japa so much better than spoken? John Woodroffe comments: "where there is audible utterance the mind thinks of the words and the process of correct utterance, and is therefore to a greater . . . or less degree . . . distracted from a fixed attention to the meaning of the mantra."[14] Finally, japa culminates in "*ajapa* where *Japa* goes on spontaneously without any physical and psychical efforts."[15] Does this close the book on japa? No, there's more.

The just mentioned SSP seems to contradict the BYY on the Self-transformative efficacy of japa. We're informed that the *parama-pada*, the "highest state," isn't realized by the practice of asana, proper diet, pranayama, silence, freedom from passion, austerities, meditation, pilgrimage, worship and devotion, "or by other means and efforts," including japa. After we've discarded all these physical practices, we're sent to "seek refuge" in the immaterial paramapada, which we then reach through the teaching and empowering word (*vanmatra*), touch (*shaktipat*), or glance (*drikpata*) of the guru.[16] Once again we see the how utterly essential the guru is in traditional yoga. We can neither start nor complete our practice without one guiding us.

▸ ▸ BEHIND THE NUMBERS

How Much Japa?

Do you have some extra time on your hands and yearn to achieve liberation? Japa might be the way to go. According to the SS, by repeating your mantra one lakh times, you'll become sexually irresistible. Two lakh times will change you into a place of pilgrimage—people will leave their families for you, travel hundreds of miles, give you all their property, and succumb to your power. Three lakh times of repeating your mantra will lead your state's governor to be the next to fall under your thumb, and with six lakh, the president will join your governor, along with "his dependents, his troops, and his vehicles." Twelve lakh get you control over an assortment of demons and snakes, and 15 lakh add various adepts and heavenly creatures to your growing menagerie, as well as conferring on you long-distance hearing, clairvoyance, and omniscience.

Enough? Hardly. Eighteen lakh repetitions earn you a divine body and the ability to wander freely through the universe; 28 lakh and you can assume any form you wish; 30 lakh and you become the equal of Brahma and Vishnu; 60 lakh lift you on par with Rudra (i.e., Shiva); and 80 lakh bring you to Shakti. Finally, with one crore of repetitions, you're absorbed into the Absolute.[17]

All well and good, but before you expectantly begin your japa practice, I think you should know a lakh equals 100,000. So let's see: 100,000 reps at one second each, without stopping to eat, sleep, or anything else will take about 70 days. Or more reasonably, if we treat this practice like a regular job—except if you're a yoga teacher—with eight-hour days, and we go straight through with no lunch or bathroom breaks, you'll need 208 days, a little more than half a year. Not too bad. Of course, to reach Shakti equivalence with eight-hour shifts, you'll need 45 years, no days off and no vacations. And oh yes, a crore equals 100 lakh, so that's 10,000,000, which means the Absolute will have to wait for you for almost 57 years. The BYY points out that japa done to the "extent of crores brings prosperity"; however, the text fails to specify what prosperity means, except to say it's called *ananta*, "endless," so whatever it is, there will apparently be an endless supply.[18] The text calls such a person a "great rarity," another one of those wonderful yoga understatements.[19]

◂ ◂

MANTRA YOGA AND ITS 16 LIMBS

mantra (from *man*, "thought," *tra*, "instrument"), "instrument of thought . . . ; a sacred formula addressed to any individual deity (e.g., *om shivaya namah*); a mystical verse or magical formula . . . , incantation, charm, spell (especially in modern times employed by the Shaktas to acquire superhuman powers; the primary Mantras held to be 70 millions in number and the secondary innumerable).

Monier Monier-Williams, *The Sanskrit-English Dictionary*

I imagine most of us are familiar with mantras from our classes. Many teachers like to begin and/or end their classes with some kind of a group-recited mantra—three OMs seem to be popular—and maybe a short acknowledgment of a favored deity, like the Shiva mantra in the epigraph. But there's far more to Mantra Yoga than this, surprisingly so. The practice actually consists of 16 limbs, more than any other yoga practice I've been able to find:[20]

1. Devotion (*bhakti*) is defined as "exclusive attachment toward one's worshipped deity."[21]

2. Purification (*shuddhi*) of the body (*kaya*) and mind (manas) is conducted in a proper environment (*sthana*)—e.g., either under one of five preferred trees; in a cow pen, a guru's house, a temple, a forest; at a sacred river crossing (*tirtha*)—and facing in the right direction (*dik*), either east or north.

3. Seat (*asana*) is a sitting pose appropriate for meditation, of which only two are accepted in this school: Lotus Pose (*padmasana*) and Auspicious Pose (*svastikasana*).

4. "Serving the five limbs" (*pancanga sevana*) includes daily reading of the BG; reciting the "thousand names of the deity" (*sahasranama*); singing songs of praise (*stava*); wearing an amulet for protection (*kavaca*); and "heart" opening (*hridaya*) practice.

5. Conduct (*acara*) is adherence to a very detailed set of behavioral rules.

6. Concentration (*dharana*).

7. "Serving the divine space" (*divya desha sevana*) is compared to "milk pervading the entire body of a cow." As the milk "comes out only through her udder, so also the Supreme Atma, though all-pervasive, develops only in the Divya-desha," a consecrated space.[22]

8. Pranayama.

9. Mudra is said to "please the deities." Though not explained in the text, this likely refers to the folk etymology of the word, which is *mud*, meaning "to be happy." There are 19 hand mudras approved for the worship of Vishnu, 10 for Mahadeva (Shiva), one for the sun, seven for Ganesha, and nine for Durga. The list continues with mudras commemorating female deities like Lakshmi, Sarasvati, and Tara.

10 and 11. There are two libations for the deities: "satiating" (*tarpana*), a libation of water mixed with various substances and other fluids, such as honey, camphor, and ghee; and *havana*, a libation of fire.

12. Offering (*bali*) to the deity, the "best" of which is *atmabali*, "offering one's own self."[23]

13. There are two kinds of sacrifice (*yaga*), internal and external, the "glory" of the former is "above all."[24]

14. Japa is the "repeated utterance or recitation of a Mantra according to certain rules."[25]

15. Meditation (*dhyana*), which is alone the "cause of knowledge and emancipation."[26]

16. Samadhi of Mantra Yoga is called the "great being" (*maha bhava*), which is the "supreme objective" of this school.

▸ ▸ BEHIND THE NUMBERS

How Many Mantras Are There?
What Are Mantras Used For?

I think most everyone will agree that 35,000,000 mantras are sufficient. But just in case that's not enough for you, the same text numbers mantras at seven *koti*, and since a *koti* equals 10,000,000, that means there are 70,000,000 mantras.

Enough?

No?

Then it's said that these 70,000,000 are the main mantras, and the so-called secondary mantras are endless.

◂ ◂

It might come as something of a shock to learn we can use a mantra to settle a score with an enemy. That seems at best very unyogic, no matter how much they might deserve it. But in fact, mantras are used for many reasons other than to worship or communicate with a deity. They can also be invoked, among other things, to acquire superhuman powers, communicate with ghosts and shoo away evil influences and devils, cure disease, and control others' thoughts and actions. Mantra apparently has as many uses as a Swiss Army knife. "From the mother's womb to the funeral pyre a Hindu literally lives and dies in Mantra."[27]

In the end, the most important factor in the efficacy of the mantra is the chanter's character. A good person, who has sincere faith in Shiva and follows all the mandated daily rituals, will reap the many benefits that accrue from this mantra. But even someone who's not especially decent, faithful, and devout, will nonetheless be rewarded in some small way.

▸ ▸ BEHIND THE NUMBERS

16 in Sanskrit

The Sanskrit word for 16 is *shodashan, shodasha* in compounds. One unusual meaning is the "length of the sixteenth of a man," which is, according to the dictionary, said of a brick.

Before I began research for this book in earnest, of all the numbers I finally included, I was by far the least aware of the number 16. It turns out though, according to Jan Gonda, that there's a "vast amount of material on the dominance of the number 16 in Indian culture."[28] Gonda believes that 16's prevalence derives from its association with Prajapati who, as "lord of the creatures," presides over procreation and represents the All, the Totality.[29] Alain Danielou echoes this sentiment, writing that 16 is the number "taken to represent perfection, totality."[30]

Gonda locates the earliest appearance of this link between Prajapati and 16 (*shodashi*) in the White Yajur Veda, composed sometime before 600 BCE:

> Than whom there is none other born more mighty, who has pervaded all existing creatures—Prajapati, rejoicing in his offspring, he, Shodashi, maintains the three great lustres (i.e., Sun, lightning, fire).[31]

This association of 16 with Prajapati, Gonda continues, likely influenced the doctrine of the 16 parts of Brahman, divided equally among four quarters. Each of the quarters serves as a focus for worship, and when successful, each bestows on the worshipper a particular name and power. So if we worship the four cardinal directions in one quarter, we're known as Far-Flung and we become "far-flung in this world"; with worship of Earth, the "intermediate region," the sky and the ocean, we're known as Limitless and so have "no limits" in the world; if we worship the sources of light and fire, the sun and moon, and lightning, we're known as Radiant, and we become "radiant" in the world; finally, if we worship the breath, sight, hearing, and the mind, we're known as Abode-possessing, and then we'll have an "abode in this world."[32]

Speaking of the breath, the Hatha texts occasionally call for a breathing pattern based on 16 counts. It never occurred to me before my research there was a possible deeper meaning to the number. So the inhale should be made for 16 counts, the inner retention of the breath (*antara kumbhaka*) 64 counts (16 × 4), the exhale 32 counts (16 × 2), and the outer retention (*bahya kumbhaka*) again 16 counts. This is the classic pranayama ratio of 1:4:2:1.[33]

It seems reasonable to contend that the 16 pattern is a reference to perfection, informing those in the know that breathing is a means that will help us attain this ultimate goal of our practice. On breathing, the *Hatha Tattva Kaumudi* notes that we should follow the "prescribed ratio," but doesn't say what that ratio is.[34] The same text notes we should practice 16 rounds of inhale and exhale to purify the nadis.[35]

Gonda further speculates that this idea of the 16-part Prajapati influenced another 16-part figure, the four-legged Brahman. The legs are speech, breath, sight, and hearing, and each of these legs has a "light": respectively, they are fire, wind, sun, and the quarters, and anyone who knows all four "gleams and glows with fame, glory, and the lustre of sacred knowledge."[36]

Because of our micro-macro relation to Brahman, the 16 parts of Brahman are then reflected in each of us. These parts consist of the life breath, faith, space, wind, fire, water, earth, senses, mind, and food; and from food come strength, austerity, Vedic formulas, rites, and worlds; "and in the worlds, name." Just as rivers flow to the sea and merge into it, losing their individual identities, these parts proceed toward and merge into the person, "losing their names and visible appearances," and so the person becomes "partless and immortal."[37]

Robert Hume explains that the "cosmic Person" is immanent in each of us, we are its most "distinctive manifestation." We then tend to return to, and merge into, the immortal Person, and so lose our "finite individuality."[38]

Gonda offers a long list of examples of the uses of 16 in Indian culture, not only by the Hindus, but the Buddhists too—which I won't cover. Here are just a few selections from the list.

There are 16 divine mothers,[39] and 16 offerings for worshipping the goddess: water for washing the feet, for the offering, for rinsing the mouth before eating and washing the mouth after, and for her bath; also clothes, jewels, perfume, flowers, incense sticks, lights, food, wine, *pan* (a yummy mélange of areca nut, lime, catechu, a kind of herb, cardamom, cinnamon, wrapped in betel leaf and secured with a clove), water for oblation, and obeisance.[40]

There are 16 services (*upacara*) rendered to an installed deity or idol, whether in a household shrine or public temple. These include ceremonial bathing (*snana*) of and honoring (*arcaka*) the idol, circumambulation (*pradakshina*) of the shrine, gift giving (*bali dana*), ceremonial waving (*arati*) of a lighted lamp in front of the idol, asking favors of the god by offering food (*prasada*), entreaty (*prarthana*) to the deity for favors, and dismissal (*visarjana*), saying goodbye to the deity at the end of the worship.

David Gordon White has a different take on the reason for 16's importance. He first notes though that in the Brahmanas, the priestly commentaries on Vedic ritual and symbolism, 16 was identified as Brahman which, like Prajapati, stands for the All. But even more significant than this is 16's relation to the waxing and waning of the moon. Each night of the lunar fortnight is known as a digit (*kala*, pronounced kuh-LAH), so there are 15 of these mundane digits in all. To this is added a transcendent 16th, identified with Atman and called the "deathless digit" (*amrita kala*).

During each lunar month, the moon fills up with the elixir of immortality, which it then literally rains down on the Earth, to provide the "fluid source of every creature's vitality."

Human life depends on the deathless digit, which in the microcosm is located in the cranial vault, the equal of the "single immortal lunar digit that dwells in the world on new-moon nights."[41]

There's one 16 we might not want to know about. According to Danielou, 16 years represents the "age of accomplished perfection," after which he says, "decline sets in."[42] We find such a person in the Girl-of-16 (Shodashi), who is five-faced Shiva's power and rules over all that is "perfect, complete, beautiful."[43]

▸ ▸ BEHIND THE NUMBERS

Shodashi and the Moon

Shodashi can also mean "the 16th." This is a reference to the phases of the moon, the lunar days (*tithi*), of which there are 15 in the light half of the month and 15 in the dark half, 30 in all. Shodashi is the 16th "hidden digit" of the moon, which "deliberately plays on the symbolism of 'plus one'" (see p. 97). As the 16th, she "pushes beyond the realms of ordinary reality and is identified with the achievement of ultimacy or the final goal of liberation."[44]

◂ ◂

THREE AND OM

The worlds are three in number. The Vedas are three in number. Sandhyas occur thrice. The letters are three in number (A, U, M). Fires are three in number. Gunas are three in number. All these rest on the three letters. He who knows the secret of these three letters . . . and learns from the mouth of his Guru, that it is no other than the Brahman . . . [who pervades] the entire world of phenomena in the belief "all this is I alone." That is the Truth.

Yoga Tattva Upanishad 134

It's generally agreed among scholars and teachers that OM is the root (*mula*) or seed (*bija*) mantra, the one from which all the other countless mantras are produced and into which they "ultimately dissolve."[45] Its symbol—which actually looks to us like our number 3 with a tail trailing behind and a Cheshire cat smile above that—is certainly one of the more recognizable yoga images, along with the lotus and the dancing Shiva.

Why is OM so attached to three? The number reflects the mantra's three basic elements—though to be clear, sometimes those elements are determined to be either four or five. We usually see it spelled the way it has been so far, OM. But the O is actually created in Sanskrit by a junction (*sandhya*) or blending of two vowels, *a* and *u*. This junction is internal, derived from two consecutive letters in the same word. Junctions can also be external, which is a blending between two consecutive words.

OM is known as "three syllables" (*tryakshara*, with *akshara* also meaning "imperishable," which reflects the belief that OM is eternal) in a reference to its three elements, which in turn are designated as "makers" (*kara*), *a-kara, u-kara, ma-kara*. Notice here that when transliterated to the Roman alphabet, the *m* is accompanied with an *a*. That's because like all 34 basic Sanskrit consonants, the *m* is a syllable, not a letter like our Roman alphabet's *m*. This means all of the consonants are accompanied with an inherent *a*, so that rather than being pronounced "em," as our letter is, the Sanskrit *m*—even though the *a* doesn't appear—is pronounced "muh."

As I mentioned, there are at least two dozen synonyms for OM that begin with the prefix *tri-* (or *try-* or *trir-*). For the Indians, "this whole world" is OM,[46] and its three syllables (*akshara trayam*) are the "highest domain and greatest refuge."[47] It would be hard to find any aspect of life not symbolized by an OM-based trio. It starts right at the top with the three deities (*tridaivatya*) of the Hindu's triple form (*trimurti*)—Brahma, Vishnu, Rudra (Shiva)—with their three selves (*triratma*)—strength (*bala*), power (*virya*), brilliance (*tejas*)—and their three natures (*trisvabhava*)—wisdom (*jnana*), dominion (*aishvarya*), and power (*shakti*). Next in line are the three worlds (*triravasthana*)—Earth (*bhur*), Atmosphere (*bhuvas*), and Heaven (*svar*)—three Vedas (*tribrahma*)—Rig, Sama, Yajur—the three sacrificial fires (*trimukha*), and the three purposes of daily life (*triprayojana*)—following the natural order of the universe (*dharma*), acquiring wealth (*artha*), and fulfilling desire (*kama*). The three times (*trikala*) are covered—past, present, and future—and the three genders (*trilinga*)—feminine, masculine, and neuter—the three states (*tripada*)—waking, sleep, and deep sleep—and the three mind states (*triravasthana*)—peaceful, terrible, and perplexed. The syllables even tell us the three places (*tristhana*) from where we should produce the sound of OM—beginning in the heart, then engaging the throat, and finally the palate. There are several more examples which we'll pass by.

▸ ▸ PRACTICE

Ajapa Mantra

> The song of the inner gander has a final secret to disclose. "Hamsa, ham-sa," it sings, but at the same time, "sa-'ham, sa-'ham."
> Heinrich Zimmer, *Myths and Symbols*
> *in Indian Art and Civilization*

Mantras may be endless, but there's one—or maybe two, depending—that's with us all the time, and easy to pronounce, no Sanskrit required. It's the sound of our own breath, which means that with every breath we take from the moment we're born to the day we pass on is a mantra. With each inhalation, the yogis say, we make a sibilant *sa* sound, with each exhalation, an aspirated *ha*. So these two syllables can be arranged in two ways.

The first, as we see in the epigraph from Heinrich Zimmer, is *sa'ham*. *Sa* stands for "this," and *ham* stands for *aham*, the Sanskrit pronoun "I." The meaning then is "This am I." This "I" is you—the limited you, that is, bound by Self-ignorance. "This," with a capital *T*, is your Self, your Atman. With each breath we take, we affirm and reaffirm this basic truth and identity.

The second arrangement is hamsa, often translated as "swan," though it can also be rendered (as Zimmer does) as "gander." She's at home both on the water and in the air, but bound to neither, and as our "inner gander," she is a symbol of our ever free "divine essence."[48] Again, with each breath we take, we remind ourselves of who we are beyond the limited self.

The natural sound of our breath makes this mantra, but we can amplify it during pranayama practice for three reasons: One, the way in which we effectuate the louder sound—which I'll describe shortly—naturally slows our breath, which is something we want to do for breathing practice. Two, the sound helps us monitor the even flow of the breath. Three, the sound helps us absorb our awareness in the breath.

Now inhale through your nose, open your mouth wide and exhale through your mouth. Feel where the exhale touches on the back of your throat. Repeat several times, until you're confident you have a feel for the back throat. Then both inhale and exhale through your nose, directing both breaths across the back throat. This should ideally amplify the natural sound, the arrangement of the two syllables, and so the way you interpret the mantra is up to you.

◄ ◄

FOUR GREAT SAYINGS (*MAHA VAKYA*)

Every living being longs always to be happy . . . and everyone has the greatest love for herself, which is solely due to the fact that happiness is her real nature. Hence, in order to realize that inherent and untainted happiness . . . , it is essential that she should know herself. For obtaining such knowledge the enquiry "who am I?" in quest of the self is the best means.

The Collected Works of Ramana Maharshi

The Vedic Upanishads were compiled sometime between 800 and 300 BCE. They contain a wealth of spiritual inspiration which, it's said, is summarized in about two dozen sayings (*vakya*), of which four are considered great (*maha*). Each is taken from one of the four compilations upon which the spiritual life of the Hindus is based, the *Rig, Yajur, Sama*, and AVs.

The word *upanishad* is often interpreted to mean "to sit down near," which describes how these texts were taught originally, with the student sitting near the teacher, who relayed the teaching orally. We might wonder why the teaching was presented in this way. Wouldn't it have been easier for the student to read a book, as we might do today? There's a very good reason why the student couldn't do this, and that's because writing hadn't yet developed in India and so there were no books. All the content of the Upanishads was held in the teachers' memories, so sitting near the teacher and listening to him speak was the only way for the student to learn the teaching.

But there was another reason for sitting near, and that was to prevent the teaching from being heard by noninitiates—people who hadn't been formally accepted into the teacher's orbit. And why was this? Most yoga knowledge today—that I know of—is out in the open and accessible to just about everyone. But 2,500 years ago, the teaching was considered top secret. So much so that in fact, another name for the Upanishads is *rahasya*, "secret, concealed, mysterious." The texts' secrets were revealed only to those select souls who had convinced the teacher they were ripe for instruction, apparently not an easy thing to do.

This oral tradition continued even after writing was developed, and is still in practice today. It was thought the teacher passing the inspiration orally to his students was an act that recreated the original passing of the Veda from the deity to the first seers at the beginning of the current world cycle. In this way the Veda has been handed down from one generation to the next, like a baton passed from runner to runner in a relay race, and so through time the texts have maintained their connection to the source. Because of this, the Veda is known as *shruti*, "what is heard," as opposed to *smriti*, "what is remembered," that is, texts composed by humans, which carry less authority.

Humans are a curious bunch. We've always been curious about the world around us, no doubt for practical survival reasons at first, but eventually about more philosophical things like its origin, its purpose, even its end. As time passed, and the everyday demands of survival eased a bit, we grew curious about our own beginning, purpose, and end. This naturally raised three questions: Where did I come from? What am I doing here? And where am I going? Notice the one constant in all three questions is "I." This leads to the central question about ourselves at the heart of most yoga schools that has attracted the interest of sages and thinkers for more than 2,000 years, and that is: Who am I?

It must have taken us a long time to first ask that question, and even longer to come up with an answer. Nowadays I suspect most people would think the answer is obvious. Their "I" is their *ego*, the Latin word for the pronoun *I*. My dictionary would back that answer up: the *ego* is defined as the "self of an individual."

But just as we found with the four states of consciousness, the yogis would have a much different answer. They may grant that the ego is a kind of self. But since it's limited to one individual, which means that it's necessarily limited in time, space, and capacity, it's in a constant state of flux and so changes over time, and it's subject to wild swings of emotion from uncontrolled ecstacy to debilitating depression, they say it can't possibly be our true nature. The answer to the question, the "I," can only be some existent that's not limited in any way, which means it must transcend time and space, be changeless or static, and as a consequence of both, unceasingly blissful. This of course is the Self.

Our question and its answer is at the heart of the Upanishads, and consequently of the maha vakya too, which are the essence of those texts. The four are in English:

1. Brahman is knowing (or consciousness) (*prajnanam brahma*).[49]
2. That is you (*tat tvam asi*).[50]
3. This Self is brahman (*ayam atma brahman*).[51]
4. I am Brahman (*aham brahmasmi*).[52]

The ordering you see here is a traditional four-step sequence that represents a gradual intensification of practice and understanding, from hearing, to reflection, to meditation, to liberation and the answer to our question. Let's review each step briefly, in order.

1. Since we're looking to know something about ourselves, the first vakya deals with the nature and source of knowing. This is equated with Atman/Brahman, the "two pillars on which rests nearly the whole edifice of Indian philosophy."[53]

2. The second vakya recreates the student-teacher encounter, when the teacher tells us straight out the answer to the question. Nowadays this answer is available to all and sundry; it's posted online for the world to see. To us this seems perfectly natural; after all, important information like this should have the widest possible distribution.

   But this isn't the way it worked 3,000 years ago. We should remember that originally this answer—the entire teaching in fact—was held as top secret (*rahasya*), and only the most qualified students were fortunate enough to be given this information. Everybody else—the majority of the population—were shut out of the secret. But as we all know, being told the answer is a step in the right direction, but there's still some way to go before we achieve final realization and liberation.

3. The third vakya draws the essential equivalence between the Atman, the Self of the individual, and Brahman, the Self of the world, affirming that while they appear to be separate existents, they are in fact one and the same. This brings the student to the central teaching of the Upanishads, called monism—or in Sanskrit, *advaita*, literally "not-two."

4. Finally, the fourth vakya is the crowning statement, a self-proclamation, a recognition of and total immersion in the answer to the question, which is "I am Brahman." It's important to remember here that saying "I am Brahman" is something of a double-edged sword. Taken the wrong way, it could inflate the ego and create a false sense of superiority to our world and its creatures. Be aware that here the "I" isn't the limited individual on our driver's license; rather, "I" is the limitless Self of the embodied being.

11

POWERS AND LIBERATION
BY THE NUMBERS

The liberation of that Yogin is on the palm of his hand,—of
him who meditates on the imperishable lustre of consciousness
seated in the middle of the lotus of the heart.
Trishikhi Brahmana Upanishad, mantra 156

The world of traditional yoga is home to many oddities in word and
action. But to me, nothing is odder than the supernatural powers that
are claimed to accompany an advancing practice. We might think this
is a fringe subject, that the powers only show up in a handful of obscure
texts on the outskirts of mainstream yoga literature. But we'd be wrong.
The powers are talked about everywhere, in major texts ranging from the
epic MBh to the YS to certain Puranas in the vast encyclopedic collection of olden times tales to the Yoga Upanishads. Not only that, they're
taken very seriously, as we all would, I suppose, if we were convinced
there were yogis out there with powers "so immense that a common person can't even imagine it."[1]

In Sanskrit, the powers are called *siddhis*, "accomplishments," or
more rarely *upasargas*, "troubles, misfortunes," and *vibhutis*, "mighty,
powerful." These powers are apparently a human birthright, hidden
away in our body like a flame in a log, waiting to be set free when the

yoga match is struck and applied. Most people, though, will never know what it's like to wield even the least of the powers. Only the yogis have the time and the training to coax these powers into the light of day, and even for them it's not that easy. But when they're successful and the powers kick in, watch out: they're not to be trifled with.

The primary means through which the powers are developed in Patanjali Yoga is called *samyama*, "holding together," that is, the simultaneous practice of concentration (*dharana*), meditation (*dhyana*), and samadhi, the so-called "interior limbs" (*antaranga*) and the last three of Patanjali's eight-limb discipline. In the YS, the powers are listed mostly in the third chapter, appropriately titled *Vibhuti Pada*, the "Power (*bhuti*) Chapter."

Be aware that samyama isn't the only way to generate powers. The five yamas and five niyamas[2] are each accompanied by a special power; for example, when the yogi is established in nonharming (*ahimsa*), "all enmity is abandoned in his presence."[3]

► ► BEHIND THE NUMBERS

Four Alternative Means to the Powers

This sutra opens the fourth chapter of the YS. It suggest four possible alternative ways, other than samyama and samadhi—the ways discussed in the previous chapter—to attain powers. Asceticism, which perfects the yogi's will so that they can take on "any form" or go anywhere "at will," mantra recitation, and birth are generally accepted by modern commentators. Birth here means those individuals, because of a store of good karma, who came into life as fully accomplished yogis. B.K.S. Iyengar singles out Ramakrishna Paramahamsa and Ramana Maharshi as examples.[4]

The fourth way of herbs (*oshadhi*), though, meets with some resistance, since it's assumed that this refers to something a bit more mind-altering than oregano or thyme. The effects of using herbs is either downplayed or rejected altogether. Svami Hariharananda Aranya, who knew a thing or two about asceticism—he lived alone in an artificial cave for the last 21 years of his life—adds a nice touch, writing that "Witches were supposed to practice this method."[5] Feuerstein puts his foot down, and wants nothing to do with herbs. Nowhere, he writes, in any yoga scripture "do we find the claim that drugs can replace the years of self-discipline and commitment demanded of the *yogin*."[6]

The feeling I get from the commentaries is that the powers that emerge through these means are somehow less valued and honored than those derived from samyama, especially when it comes to drugs. But it's not clear what the concern is all about, since the needed drug would seem to be extremely difficult to acquire. According to Vacaspati Mishra, when a human "for some cause or another reaches the mansions of the demons (*asura*)," they may make use of the "elixirs-of-life" offered by the "lovely damsels of the demons" and attain agelessness, deathlessness, and "other perfections."[7] Exactly where these mansions are and how to reach them isn't revealed, not that any of us would want to venture there anyway.

◂ ◂

The best known of the powers are the eight great accomplishments (*maha siddhi*), summarized in the commentaries at YS 3.45 by Vyasa (V) and Vacaspati Mishra (M). They are:

1. Minuteness (*animan*)—the power to become as small as an atom (V)
2. Magnitude (*mahiman*)—the power of unlimited expansion, to become in "dimension an elephant or a mountain or town" (M)
3. Levity (*laghiman*)—the power to decrease your weight and float in the air "like the tuft of a reed" (M)
4. Attainment (*prapti*)—the power of extension, so if standing on the Earth, you could touch the moon with the tip of your finger (M)
5. Freedom of will (*prakamya*)—the power, if you so desire, to dive into the solid earth and emerge again, "as if in water" (V)
6. Mastery (*vashitva*)—the power to master the elements and their products, and not be mastered "by others" (V)

7. Supremacy (*ishitritva*)—the power over the production, absorption, and arrangement of the traditional elements and their products (V)
8. Desire dwelling (*kama avasayiyva*)—the power to determine "things according to desire" (V)

Just as Patanjali's nine *antarayas* are the tip of the obstacle iceberg, these "great eight" are similarly the tip of the powers' iceberg. So what are these powers all about? (Note that I'm discussing mostly the powers in the YS—to include powers from other sources would make this chapter far too long.) Notice that the eight greats are powers you employ mostly to affect yourself, to make yourself smaller, bigger, stronger, lighter, and more willfully free. Notice too there's no mention here of powers to help other people, to empower the yogi to improve the lives of those around him. This wasn't, as far as I can tell, much of a concern for Patanjali's followers; they were primarily interested in freeing themselves from the grip of matter.

But the powers enumerated in YS chapter 3 have a much broader application. Indeed, a yogi with these powers is bound neither by time nor space; he can gaze into the past and future and so foretell the day of his death. He can cross great distances almost instantaneously. He's completely mastered his senses, can peer into the subtle realms, understands the "functioning of consciousness,"[8] can read other minds and inhabit other bodies, or go bodiless entirely. He can make himself as strong as an elephant, walk on water, and become invisible. And oh, he can, if he so desires, live far beyond the normal span of years. "All the powers come under his control and command. . . . He can see the entire universe like pearls kept in the palm which means he becomes . . . omniscient . . . [and] he enjoys eternity."[9]

How do our teachers and scholars make sense of these powers, if at all? Teachers are over a barrel when it comes to Patanjali. If they reject the powers, they can't escape the implication that Patanjali might have gotten other things wrong, which casts a shadow over the entire YS, not to mention all the subsequent texts that follow its teaching. Besides, we're continually told that every word in the text is there for a reason, and this must also necessarily be so for the 40 or so "power sutras" which make up 75 percent of chapter 3 and 20 percent of the text.

Carl Olson, in *Indian Asceticism: Power, Violence, and Play*, surveys the positions taken by, according to my rough count, 15 scholars, mostly from twentieth-century writing. He distributes them across a range of reactions, from highly skeptical on one end of the scale to more accepting on the opposite end. The skeptics believe the powers to be the result of hypnotism, mental illusions, and hallucinations. Others see them as "spurious aspects or magical residues" that belong to a "foundational stage" of the development of yoga,"[10] and that seem to conflict with Patanjali's rationalism. Highly regarded Indologist Gerald Larson calls the powers "imaginative fantasies."[11] He sees evidence that two sutras in chapter 3 "express a degree of skeptical caution about these powers, thereby providing some textual evidence that these experiences were not meant literally."[12]

But Olson takes issue here with Larson for not treating the powers seriously. He faults Larson for injecting his "personal skepticism into his interpretation," which he dismisses, rather condescendingly it seems to me, as "perfectly understandable for a person living in the twenty-first century" who's "far removed from the time period of the text compiled by Patanjali."[13]

The most levelheaded approach to the powers that I came across is that of Edwin Bryant in his translation/commentary of the YS. His justification is quite long and involved, and I'm not sure I can do it justice so I won't try to review it in detail here. Briefly then, he first points out four shortcomings of modern siddhis naysayers, calling what they do "reductionistic modes of interpretation." They impose "terms and categories" on the powers that are alien to the "frame of reference of the system or body of knowledge in question." In doing so, they assume "elistist perspectives" that paint the yogi as a "hapless mystic" who has no idea what's happening.

This leads to the assumption that the powers need a "specialized and 'rational' vantage point," that of the "objective" scholar, to make sense of them. And finally, the scholars don't ever consider their own limitations when considering these phenomena.[14]

Bryant then attempts to make sense of the powers by conceptualizing them "through traditional Yogic perspectives." The upshot of his argument, as I understand it, is that the yogi is able to penetrate into the subtle layers of matter and so transcend the limitations imposed by the kleshas and the ego (ahamkara). This allows the yogi to manipulate the external effects of matter. Bryant quotes at length from G. M. Koelman:

> Since *prakritic* Nature is, in its entirety, one single substance working for the liberation of the Selves, it does not seem strange that, in proportion that the *yogi* approaches the final goal, prakriti Nature looses its hold on him and he gains control over it.[15]

So most contemporary teachers and scholars more or less come out in favor of the powers, though that favor is usually based more on faith than concrete evidence. None of the pro-power advocates actually describe being in the presence of an unquestionable exhibition of any of the powers. But not all scholars are on board with this.

The manifestation of the powers is thought to be a positive, a sign your practice is progressing. If your practice is sound, writes B.K.S. Iyengar, these powers are the "effects you experience. If you don't experience any of these effects, that means your practice is imperfect."[16] I can understand how this test may apply to traditional practitioners, who spent their lives cultivating the practices that would lead to the powers. But it's absurd to expect the average modern-day student to experience anything like a power, and Iyengar, who dealt with thousands and thousands of Westerners over more than four decades, should know that better than anyone.

But once the powers do manifest, we're strongly advised by our teachers and scholars to ignore them, to put them in our back pocket and leave them there. As we know, the primary push in yoga is toward Self-realization, and the powers are viewed as tempting distractions that will divert the yogi from that goal, possibly with disastrous results. This is why the old texts continuously and emphatically insist the practice should be held in the strictest secrecy and that every candidate for instruction should be thoroughly vetted so there's no doubt about her character or intentions.

But the old texts, at least as many as I have access to, seem ambivalent about the powers. The SSP describes a yogi in the eleventh and twelfth years of practice. "In the eleventh year she becomes omniscient and gains all supernatural powers. In the twelfth year, being like Shiva, she becomes herself the creator and destroyer."[17] This doesn't sound like this yogi is holding anything back. But then we read in the HRA, "A *muni* (i.e., an ascetic who's taken a vow of silence) relinquishing attachment toward powers (*siddhis*), attains liberation during life. In the face of the exquisite Bliss, one considers siddhis as trash."[18]

But don't worry, because the universe's creator, who Vyasa names Hiranyagarbha, the "Golden Womb," anticipated the possibility of a fallen yogi. To protect creation, Hiranyagarbha established certain safeguards right in the beginning, which make it impossible for a bad apple to go against his will and upset the universal apple cart.

TWO FORMS OF LIBERATION AND THE MEANING OF ONE: ISOLATION (*KAIVALYA*) AND *MOKSHA*

The mumukshus are of two kinds: the votaries of kaivalya (Self-realization) and the votaries of moksha (release from samsara).

Yatindra Mata Dipika 8.16

As we've already established, we're all afflicted with a condition known as avidya, the mistaken belief that we are who we're not and not who we are (see p. 119). This leads to a most unpleasant case of existential suffering, for which there's only one cure: becoming who we are and letting go of who we're not, which is always easier said than done. Dying won't even get us off the hook, since if we pass away with our avidya intact, after a period of bodiless quiescence we're shuttled right back into another mortal coil, and the suffering picks up where it left off in the previous life.

Yoga offers a number of solutions to the avidya conundrum, proposing that if we assiduously follow this or that program, we just might gain liberation, though there are no money-back guarantees this will happen no matter how assiduous we are. The question now is: What is meant by *liberation*?

We've ascertained the yogis will never be praised for consistency, though the expectation for that is our issue, as overly rational Westerners, not theirs. As the American transcendentalist Ralph Waldo Emerson once opined, "A foolish consistency is the hobgoblin of little minds." The universe presents us with an indeterminate number of mysteries, some which we may expect someday to solve, others maybe never. As the Shatapatha Brahmana reminds us, the "gods love the mystic."[19]

So then we shouldn't be surprised that there are different ideas about just what liberation means. There are two in particular that could hardly be more dissimilar. On one side is that championed by our friend Patanjali. His form of liberation results in two things of equal importance. One, it results in a complete withdrawal of the Self (*purusha*) from its problematic connection with matter (prakriti). Then, says Patanjali, the Self abides in its own form (*svarupa*) or essence. It's important to understand here that it's not the Self that's actually liberated, because in effect it was never really bound. It's that little bit of matter we so lovingly think of as "my body" that's released, recycled to the great storehouse of *pradhana* ("primary germ"), the primal matter and source of the universe. It's never been clear to me who or what in this system suffers. It doesn't seem like it's the insentient material body, since lacking intelligence it can't feel; nor does it seem to be the sentient immaterial Self, since it has nothing to feel with. The contradictions in Patanjali's system are difficult to resolve and accept. The yogis may not be consistent *between* systems, but *within* each system they're usually completely rational.

The second consequence of Patanjali's liberation is that the Self figuratively dismounts the painted avidya pony that it was riding on the un-merry-go-round of continual rebirth. It will never again suffer through another embodiment, never again be subject to the slings and arrows of outrageous fortune. This dual escape from prakriti and punar janman (see p. 133) is Patanjali's liberation, kaivalya or "perfect isolation," from *kevala*, "alone."

We might ask: what is it like to be in kaivalya? And the answer is: it's hard to say. Kaivalya's not an experience that can be described in words; consequently, most books on Patanjali Yoga haven't much to say about it. Mircea Eliade writes that kaivalya isn't "absolute emptiness," but rather a "total absence of objects in consciousness" which is "saturated with a direct and total intuition of being." It's a state "without sensory content or intellectual structure, an unconditioned state that is no longer 'experience' . . . but 'revelation.'"[20]

▸ ▸ BEHIND THE NUMBERS

Two Forms of Mukti: Videh a *(Bodiless)* and Jivan *("Keep Alive")*

Patanjali's form of liberation is also known as videha mukti, "bodiless liberation." In order to be fully liberated, the purusha must sever all ties with prakriti; in other words, it must exit the body (*vi*, "away from," *deha*, "body"). To us, captives as we are of avidya, dropping the body like that would be called "death." Of course, from a yogi's perspective, getting free of prakriti is the whole point of the practice.

There's a second kind of mukti, which we'll look at shortly. This is jivan mukti, liberated while living (from *jiv*, "to live, be or remain alive"). It represents an entirely different attitude toward the body and the world, one that fits in well with modern yoga.

◂ ◂

There's some speculation about what happens to the purusha post-kaivalya. One belief is that each Self is a self-enclosed monad. About this Haridas Bhattacharyya comments that the final state is "complete freedom from material contact and no communion of any kind with any other released soul."²¹ Feuerstein once suggested to me that since all the purushas were ultimately identical, they may all gather together in the great by-and-by and spend forever in blissful community.

This is how Patanjali interprets "one." The Self is stripped of everything that outwardly makes it human, since that humanity is highly undesirable. But if we enter the Tantric world, everything radically changes, though there's still that bothersome confusion about our true identity.

Patanjali's world is essentially like that bunny with the bass drum in the commercial for batteries, it's a windup mechanism that just keeps going and going with only one purpose: to provide for the liberation of individual purushas. Once that happens, its function is fulfilled and it's shuffled off to pradhana. The Tantric world—which for all intents and purposes is also that of Hatha Yoga—is the creation of the goddess Shakti. She's both the material and efficient cause of our world; in other words, she shapes our world—and our body—from the stuff of her own body, in which we are embedded. The human body now is the "most important" of 8.4 million "bodily forms," because it's in this form and no other that we get "knowledge of the Essence."²² We should then all make "persistent efforts" to preserve this "precious wealth" of the body.²³ It's said in this regard that there's no liberation without practice, and there's no practice without a human body. Needless to say, this represents a revolutionary revaluation of the body.

The practitioner's goal now is *moksha*, a most interesting word. Not only does it mean "liberation," but also "settling a question" (which suggests that of our true identity) and "discharge of a debt" (which suggests a payoff of our karmic debt). In Patanjali's world, when we finally realize the truth about ourselves, it results in a total separation from the material world. In the Tantric world when we realize our true Self, it results in a union not only with Shiva-Shakti, but since the universe is the body of the goddess, with that universe itself. Where Patanjali's one equals a single, isolated monad, the Tantric one equals everything, an all-encompassing union.

Notes

1. ZERO (THE VOID) BY THE NUMBERS

1. Georges Ifrah, trans. by David Bellos, E. F. Harding, Sophie Wood, and Ian Monk, *The Universal History of Numbers* (New York: John Wiley & Sons, Inc., 2000), 438.
2. Troy Wilson Organ, *Western Approaches to Eastern Philosophy* (Athens, Ohio: Ohio University Press, 1975), 24.
3. Betty Heimann, *Facets of Indian Thought* (New York: Schocken Books, 1964), 98.
4. Alex Bellos, 7 October 2013, *Guardian.* www.theguardian.com/science/.
5. Heinrich Zimmer, ed. Joseph Campbell, *Philosophies of India* (Princeton, NJ: Princeton University Press, 1971), 75.
6. DU 60–62.
7. DU 7.
8. YSU 4.18.
9. Karl H. Potter, ed., *Encyclopedia of Indian Philosophies*, vol. 3: Advaita Vedanta up to Shankara and His Pupils (Delhi: Motilal Banarsidass, 1981), 76.
10. VS 1.1.2.
11. Shankara in his commentary on VS 2.1.34.
12. M. Hiriyanna, *Outlines of Indian Philosophy* (London: George Allen & Unwin, 1970), p. 54.
13. William Mahoney, *The Artful Universe: An Introduction to the Vedic Religious Imagination* (Albany: State University of New York Press, 1998), p. 227.
14. Pashupata Brahmana Upanishad, Purva Kanda 11.

2. INDIAN PHILOSOPHY BY THE NUMBERS

1. KT 9.15.
2. Paul Deussen, trans., "Prana Agni Hotra 4," in *Sixty Upanishads of the Veda*, vol. 2 (Delhi: Motilal Banarsidass, 1980), p. 650.
3. Mircea Eliade, *Yoga: Immortality and Freedom* (Princeton, NJ: Princeton University Press, 1973), 3.
4. GS 1.6–7.
5. KU 6.11, translation by Patrick Olivelle.
6. *Karikas* on the MuU, *prakarana* 2.
7. BG 13.30.
8. VS 3.9.
9. SSP 6.38.
10. YS 1.21–22.
11. ATU 18.
12. Georg Feuerstein, *Textbook of Yoga* (London: Rider, 1975), 144.
13. Edwin F. Bryant, *The Yoga Sutras of Patanjali* (New York: North Point Press, 2009), xliii.
14. Georg Feuerstein, *The Philosophy of Classical Yoga* (Rochester, VT: Inner Traditions International, 1996), 24.
15. Gerald James Larson and Ram Shankar Bhattacharya, eds., *Encyclopedia of Indian Philosophies: Yoga: India's Philosophy of Meditation*, vol. 12 (Delhi: Motilal Banarsidass, 2008), 29.
16. Georg Feuerstein, *Wholeness or Transcendence? Ancient Lessons for the Emerging Global Civilization* (Burdett, NY: Larson Publications, 1992), 191.
17. YS 2.18.
18. YS 4.32.

3. THE YOGA WORLD BY THE NUMBERS

1. *Pratya Bhijna Hridayam*, commentary on sutra 4.
2. AV 15.14–18.
3. SSP 3.13.
4. SSP 3.14.
5. Samkhya Karika 12.
6. YS 2.41.
7. Arthur Avalon, *Tantra of the Great Liberation* (*Mahanirvana Tantra*) (New York: Dover Publications, 1972), xlvi.

8. Avalon, *Tantra of the Great Liberation*, xlvi.

9. RV 10.34.

10. Cornelia Dimmitt and J.A.B. van Buitenen, ed. and trans., *Classical Hindu Mythology: A Reader in the Sanskrit Puranas* (Philadelphia: Temple University Press, 1978), 40.

11. MNT 21–29.

12. Dimmitt and van Buitenen, *Classical Hindu Mythology*, 22.

13. MNT 37–50.

14. See YS 2.51.

15. John Grimes, *A Concise Dictionary of Indian Philosophy* (Albany, NY: State University of New York Press, 1996), 103.

4. SHIVA AND SHAKTI BY THE NUMBERS

1. Rudra Samhita: Parvarti Khanda, 19.15–17.

2. Ananda Coomaraswamy, *The Dance of Shiva* (New York: The Noonday Press, 1957), 79.

3. BG 13.34.

4. Dolf Hartsuiker, *Sadhus: Holy Men of India* (New York: Thames & Hudson, 1993), 22.

5. Hartsuiker, *Sadhus*, 22.

6. Hartsuiker, *Sadhus*, 22.

7. Stella Kramrisch, *The Presence of Shiva* (Princeton, NJ: Princeton University Press, 1981), 182.

8. Svacchanda Tantra 1.3.

9. MaiU 5.2.

10. Rene Guenon, *The Great Triad* (Cambridge: Quinta Essentia, 1991), 11.

11. Alain Danielou, *The Gods of India* (New York: Inner Traditions International, 1985), 24n7.

12. Kamalakar Mishra, *Kashmir Saivism: The Central Philosophy of Tantrism* (Varanasi: Indica Books, 2011), p. 197.

13. Paul Eduardo Muller-Ortega, *The Triadic Heart of Siva: Kaula Tantrism of Abhinavagupta in the Non-Dual Shaivism of Kashmir* (Albany: State University of New York Press, 1989), p. 139.

14. Kramrisch, *The Presence of Shiva*, 440.

15. Heinrich Zimmer, edited by Joseph Campbell, *Myths and Symbols in Indian Art and Civilization* (Princeton, NJ: Princeton University Press, 1972), 152.

16. Zimmer and Campbell, *Myths and Symbols,* 1532.

17. Coomaraswamy, *The Dance of Shiva,* 71.

18. Mark S. G. Dyczkowski, *The Doctrine of Vibration: An Analysis of the Doctrines and Practices of Kashmir Shaivism* (Albany, NY: State University of New York Press, 1987), 165.

19. KT 17.32.

20. SSP 4.3–8.

21. Akshaya Kumar Banerjea, *Philosophy of Gorakhnath* (Delhi: Motilal Banarsidass, 1983), 81.

22. Banerjea, *Philosophy of Gorakhnath,* 86.

23. Banerjea, *Philosophy of Gorakhnath,* 86.

24. Kamalakar Mishra, *Kashmir Shaivism: The Central Philosophy of Tantrism* (Varanasi: Indica Books, 2011), 179.

25. Mishra, *Kashmir Shaivism,* 179.

26. VS 4.5.

27. Vettam Mani, *Puranic Encyclopedia* (Delhi: Motilal Banarsidass, 1975), 216–17.

28. BVU 36–43.

29. See for example, *Trisikhi Brahmana Upanishad,* mantra 133–145; DU 7.1–6; DBU 94–106; *Yoga Tattva Upanishad* 84–104; YSU 5.29–35; GS 3.57-63; VS 4.1–16.

30. GS 3.62.

31. YSU 29–35.

5. SUBTLE BODY BY THE NUMBERS

1. Lama Anagarika Govinda, *Foundations of Tibetan Mysticism* (Bombay: B.I. Publications, 1977), 148.

2. Shankara, translated by Swami Prabhavananda and Christopher Isherwood, *Crest-Jewel of Discrimination* (*Viveka Cudamani*) (New York: New American Library, 1947), 56.

3. Shankara, *Crest-Jewel of Discrimination,* 64.

4. *Pancadasi* 3.3.

5. *Pancadasi* 3.5.

6. *Pancadasi* 3.6.

7. *Pancadasi* 3.7.

8. *Pancadasi* 3.10.

9. YCU 14.

10. Joseph Campbell, *The Masks of God: Oriental Mythology* (New York: Viking Press, 1969), 200.

11. TBU 66–76.

12. YY 4.44.

13. YY 4.46.

14. Rajiv Malhotra and Satyanarayana Dasa Babaji, *Sanskrit Non-Translatables: The Importance of Sanskritizing English* (New Delhi: Manjul Publishing House, 2020), 123.

15. N. C. Panda, *The Vibrating Universe* (Delhi: Motilal Banarsidass. 1995), 9.

16. KJN 10.9–32.

17. SSP 2.31.

18. Banerjea, *Philosophy of Gorakhnath*, 170.

19. HYP 1.15–16.

20. Grimes, *A Concise Dictionary of Indian Philosophy*, 240.

21. CU 7.3.3.

22. CU 7.26.2.

23. KU 6.15.

24. MuU 2.1.10.

25. MuU 2.2.7–8.

26. John Woodroffe, *The Serpent Power* (Madras: Ganesh, 1964), 126.

27. Woodroffe, *The Serpent Power*, 31.

28. Govinda, *Foundations of Tibetan Mysticism*, 169.

29. Govinda, *Foundations of Tibetan Mysticism*, 170.

30. Woodroffe, *The Serpent Power*, 221.

31. Ajit Mookerjee, *Kundalini: The Arousal of the Inner Energy* (Rochester, VT: Destiny Books, 1989), 53.

32. RV 7.95.1.

33. Gavin Flood, *Introduction to Hinduism* (Cambridge: University of Cambridge, 1996), 85.

34. DU 4.48–56.

35. BG 15.10.

36. SCN 32.

37. SCN 34.

38. YSU 41–46.

6. HATHA YOGA BY THE NUMBERS

1. SS 5.18.

2. SS 5.14–15.

3. See YS 2.48.

4. See the GG 1.33–34; also the KT 17.7 and ATU 16.

5. GG 1.35.

6. GG 1.36.

7. Zimmer, *Philosophies of India*, 346.

8. Knut Jacobsen, "Introduction: Yoga Traditions," in *Theory and Practice of Yoga*, Knut Jacobsen, ed. (Delhi: Motilal Banarsidass, 2008), 22.

9. BVU 51–53.

10. KT 13.128

11. J. Krishnamurti, *The First and Last Freedom* (Wheaton, IL: A Quest Book, 1954), 151, 153.

12. KT 13.57 ff.

13. KT 13.67.

14. Manu 2.201.

15. SSP 5.68–69.

16. AV 11.5.3.

17. Mircea Eliade, ed. Wendell Beane and William Doty, *Myths, Rites, and Symbols,* vol. 1 (New York: Harper & Row, 1976), p. 169.

18. KT 14.12.

19. KT 13.3–22.

20. HYP 1.1.

21. HTK 1.1 and HRA 1.1.

22. Zimmer, *Philosophies of India,* 57.

23. HYP 1.11.

24. Gavin Flood, *The Tantric Body: The Secret Tradition of Hindu Religion* (London: I. B. Taurus, 2006), 133.

25. KT 14.45.

26. KT 14.35.

27. KT 14.55.

28. HYP 4.65–68).

29. HYP 4.80–102, 105.

30. HYP 4.77.

7. PRELIMINARY PRACTICES BY THE NUMBERS

1. Patrick Olivelle, trans., *The Ashrama System: The History and Hermeneutics of a Religious Institution* (New Delhi: Munshiram Manoharlal, 1993), 223.

2. Jaideva Singh, trans., *Pratyabhijnahrdayam* (Delhi: Motilal Banarsidass, 1963), 150, n153.

3. See YS 1.2.

4. J. Krishnamurti, *The First and Last Freedom* (Wheaton, IL: Theosophical Publishing House, 1954), p. 97

5. YS, see 2.29.

6. G. A. Gaskell, *Dictionary of All Scriptures and Myths* (New York: Julian Press, 1960), 679.

7. Gaskell, *Dictionary of All Scriptures,* 245.

8. *Vayu Purana* 10.70–71.

9. Somadeva Vasudeva, trans., *The Yoga of the Malinivijayottaratantra* (Pondichery: Institut Français de Pondichery, 2004), 367.

10. Swami Ashokananda, *Avadhuta Gita of Dattatreya* (Madras: Sri Ramakrishna Math, nd), v.

11. *Avadhuta Gita* 1.48.

12. DBU 41, YCU 2, and GS 1.4.

13. MaiU 4.18 and Amrita Nada Upanishad 6.

14. GS 1.9.

15. TBU 1.15–16.

16. Mishra, *Kashmir Shaivism,* 414.

17. J. N. Mohanty, *Classical Indian Philosophy* (Lanham, MD: Rowman & Littlefield, 2000), 31.

18. SU 1.1.13.

19. See YS 1.33.

20. SU 1.2.11.

21. See SSP 2.32.

22. Haridas Bhattacharyya, ed., *The Cultural Heritage of India,* The Early Phases, vol. 1 (Calcutta: Ramakrishna Mission Institute of Culture, 1958), 13.

23. Bhattacharyya, *The Cultural Heritage of India,* 13.

24. Bhattacharyya, *The Cultural Heritage of India,* 13.

25. B.K.S. Iyengar, *The Tree of Yoga* (Boston: Shambhala Publications, 1989), 138.

26. GS, see 1.10–58.

27. Gopi Krishna, *Kundalini: The Evolutionary Energy in Man* (Berkeley, CA: Shambhala Publications, 1971), 12.

28. HYP 1.21.

29. See HYP 1.11.

30. GS 1.47.

31. GS 1.33–34.

32. Shyam Ghosh, *The Original Yoga* (New Delhi: Munshiram Manoharlal, 2004), 109.

33. *Shiva Svarodaya* 136, 138.

34. Rai Bahadur Srira Chandra Vidyarnava, *The Daily Practice of the Hindus* (Delhi: Oriental Books Reprint Corporation, 1979), 32.

35. SS 3.25, 26.

36. SS 3.25.

37. HYP 2.11.

38. GS 5.88.

8. STAGES AND OBSTACLES BY THE NUMBERS

1. YS 1.1.

2. YS 1.1.

3. YS 1.1.

4. YS 2.5.

5. YS 2.5.

6. YS 2.7.

7. YS 2.8.

8. YS 2.9.

9. BG 7.3.

10. See 1.29–30.

11. Vyasa commentary on YS 1.30.

12. YS 1.8.

13. YS 3.16.

14. YS 3.22.

15. TBU, mantra, 119–129.

16. *Bhagavata Purana* 7.5.23–24.

17. Aranaya Kanda 35–36.

18. *Vasishtha Yoga*, "The Story of the Sons of Indu" 116–17; all subsequent quotes in this section from these two verses, unless otherwise noted.

19. K. Narayanaswami Aiyer, *Laghu Yoga Vasistha* (Madras: Hoe, 1914), 235.

20. Aiyer, LYV, 235.

21. Aiyer, LYV, 235–36.

22. YS 4.7

23. YS 2.15.

24. KT 1.13–14.

25. Christopher Chapple, *Karma and Creativity* (Albany, NY: State University of New York Press, 1986), 115n1.

26. Chapple, *Karma and Creativity*, 115n1.

9. MAIN PRACTICES BY THE NUMBERS

1. SU 1.8.1.
2. GS 2.2.
3. HYP 1.44–49.
4. HYP 2.48.
5. HYP 1.53–54.
6. HYP 1.50–52.
7. HYP 1.35.
8. Shashibhusan Dasgupta, *Obscure Religious Cults* (Calcutta: Firma KLM, 1995), 204.
9. MaiU 3.3.
10. Gudrun Bühnemann, *Eighty-four Asanas in Yoga: A Survey of Traditions* (New Delhi: D. K. Printworld, 2011), 27.
11. Matthew Kapstein, "King Kunji's Banquet," in David Gordon White, ed., *Tantra in Practice* (Princeton, NJ: Princeton University Press, 2000), 54–55.
12. HYP 1.5–9.
13. Ajit Mookerjee and Madhu Khanna, *The Tantric Way* (London: Thames and Hudson, 1977), 141.
14. Cain and Revital Carroll, *Mudras of India: A Comprehensive Guide to the Hand Gestures of Yoga and Indian Dance* (London: Singing Dragon, 2012), 19.
15. Arthur Avalon (Sir John Woodroffe), trans., *Tantra of the Great Liberation (Maha Nirvana Tantra)* (New York: Dover Publications, 1972), xcv.
16. Benjamin Walker, *The Hindu World: An Encyclopedic Survey of Hinduism*, vol. 2 (New York: Frederick A. Praeger, 1969), 85.
17. KT 17.57.
18. Carrolls, *Mudras of India*, 100.
19. Carrolls, *Mudras of India*, 77.
20. GS 1.2.
21. HYP 2.69.
22. HYP 2.70.
23. HYP 2.73.
24. YS 2.51.

25. Yogi Pranavananda, trans., *Pure Yoga* (Delhi: Motilal Banarsidass, 1992), 117.

26. M.L. Gharote, Parimal Devnath, Vijay Kant Jha, eds., *Hatharatnavali* (Lonavla, India: Lonavla Yoga Institute, 2002), 51.

27. See YS 2.54.

28. SU 1.8.1; cf. VS 3.59; YY 7.4. 2.11.

29. TBU 1.34.

30. Tiru Mantiram 587.

31. DU 7.3.

32. DU 7.5.

33. DU 8.14.

34. *Muktipa Upanishad* 1.30–39.

35. Paramarthasara 78.

36. George Briggs, *Gorakhnath and the Kanphata Yogis* (1938), 13–14.

37. Fredrick Bunce, *Numbers: Their Iconographic Consideration in Buddhist & Hindu Practices* (New Delhi: D.K. Printworld, 2002), 47.

38. Bunce, *Numbers,* 47.

39. Rev. Ebenezer Burgess, trans., *Surya Siddhanta: A Textbook of Hindu Astronomy* (New Haven, CT: American Oriental Society, 1890), 39.

10. MANTRA BY THE NUMBERS

1. Jaideva Singh, trans., *Pratyabhijnahrdayam* (Delhi: Motilal Banarsidass, 1963), 135, nn74–75.

2. YSU 3.4.

3. YSU 3.4.

4. YSU 3.5.

5. Yoga Kundali Upanishad 3.18–21.

6. YY 2.15–18.

7. BYY 7.132.

8. See for example, DU 2.2.

9. HRA 3.4.

10. BYY 7.134.

11. DU 2.12–16.

12. BYY 7.141.

13. SSP 5.14.

14. Avalon, *Tantra of the Great Liberation,* cii.

15. Manoranjan Basu, *Fundamentals of the Philosophy of the Tantras* (Calcutta: Mira Basu, 1986), 479.

16. SS 5.55–59.
17. SS 5.238–51.
18. BYY 7.138.
19. SS 5.251.
20. All quotes from MYS.
21. MYS 32.
22. MYS 47.
23. MYS 56.
24. MYS 57.
25. MYS 64.
26. MYS 80.
27. John Woodroffe, *Principles of Tantra*, Part 2 (Madras: Ganesh, 1978), 58.
28. J. Gonda, *Change and Continuity in Indian Religion* (New Delhi: Munshiram Manoharlal, 1997), 115.
29. Gonda, *Change and Continuity*, 121.
30. Danielou, *The Gods of India*, 278.
31. White Yajur Veda 8.36.
32. CU 4.4–9.
33. See GS 5.39–44; VS 3.10–17.
34. HTK 36.44.
35. HTK 36.48.
36. CU 3.18.
37. See Prashna Upanishad 6.2–5.
38. Robert E. Hume, *The Thirteen Principal Upanishads* (London: Oxford University Press, 1979), 389n.
39. MNT 9.87; 10.127.
40. MNT 6.77.
41. David Gordon White, *The Alchemical Body: Siddha Traditions in Medieval India* (Chicago: University of Chicago Press, 1996), 38.
42. Danielou, *The Gods of India*, 278.
43. Danielou, *The Gods of India*, 278.
44. Douglas Renfrew Brooks, *Auspicious Wisdom: The Texts and Traditions of Srividya Sakta Tantrism in South India* (Albany, NY: State University of New York Press, 1992), 107.
45. BYY 2.1.
46. MaiU 1.
47. BYY 2.71.
48. Zimmer, *Myths and Symbols in Indian Art and Civilization*, 48–49.

49. *Aitareya Upanishad* 3.5.3.

50. CU 6.8.7.

51. MU 2.

52. *Brihad Aranyaka Upanishad* 1.4.10.

53. M. Hiriyanna, *Outlines of Indian Philosophy* (London: George Allen & Unwin, 1970), 54.

11. POWERS AND LIBERATION BY THE NUMBERS

1. *Yoga Bija* 54.

2. YS 2.29–2.45.

3. YS 2.35.

4. B.K.S. Iyengar, *Light on the Yoga Sutras of Patanjali* (London: Aquarian Press, 1993), 230.

5. Swami Hariharananda Aranya, *Yoga Philosophy of Patanjali* (Albany, NY: State University of New York Press, 1983), 347.

6. Georg Feuerstein, *The Yoga-Sutra of Patanjali* (Rochester, VT: Inner Traditions International, 1979), 126.

7. YS 4.1

8. YS 3.34.

9. AY 1.92–95.

10. Carl Olson, *Indian Asceticism: Power, Violence, and Play* (Oxford: Oxford University Press, 2015), 32.

11. Olson, *Indian Asceticism*, 33.

12. Olson, *Indian Asceticism*, 33.

13. Olson, *Indian Asceticism*, 33.

14. Bryant, *The Yoga Sutras of Patanjali*, 330.

15. Bryant, *The Yoga Sutras of Patanjali*, 337.

16. Iyengar, *Tree of Yoga*, 122.

17. SSP 5.40.

18. HRA 46.58.

19. Shatapatha Brahama 6.1.1.11.

20. Eliade, *Yoga: Immortality and Freedom*, 93.

21. Haridas Bhattacharyya, ed., *The Cultural Heritage of India*, The Philosophies, vol. 3 (Calcutta: Ramakrishna Mission Institute of Culture, 1958), 53.

22. KT 1.13.

23. KT 1.18.

Index

death, 112, 126–27, 180–81, 182
deathless digit (*amrita kala*),
166–67
Deeper Dimensions of Yoga, The
(Feuerstein), 15
deities
cakras and, 69
five, 58
five female, 58
and humans, gap between, 31–32
iconography of, 46, 47–48
six steps in approaching, 72
16 services rendered to, 166
desire (*raga*), 55, 63, 64, 101, 121,
131, 148
desire/will (*iccha*), 48
determinism, 55
Deussen, Paul, 18
devotion, 21, 72, 86, 102, 105, 128,
160, 162
dharma
attitude of, 130
cosmic and individual, 131
Dhritarashtra, 65
Dhyana Bindu Upanishad, 104
dice, 41, 42
Dictionary of All Scriptures, The, 102
*Dictionary of Imaginary Places,
The*, 33
diet and nutrition, 73, 108, 139, 158
dispassion (*vairagya*), 98, 100, 101
divine eye/sight, 78–79, 113
Doctrine of Vibration, The
(Dyczkowski), 54
Dohakosha (Saraha), 76
dualism, 15, 30
basic, 25, 27
common sense of, 16

and other systems, contrasts
between, 31
See also Patanjali Yoga
Durga, 58
Dvapara Yuga, 42, 43

ego, 101, 129, 157, 172, 173, 179. *See also*
I-am-ness
eight-limb (*ashtanga*) discipline,
102–3, 137, 146
allegorical, 105–6
alternatives to, 107
interior limbs of, 175
process of, 117
Eighty-four Asanas in Yoga
(Bühnemann), 140
elements, meditation on, 59
Eliade, Mircea, 19. See also *Myths,
Rites, Symbols*
elixir of immortality, 144–45, 166
Emerson, Ralph Waldo, 181
Encyclopaedia of Traditional Asana,
139–40
energy channels (*nadi*), 36, 74
names of ten major, 65
number of, variant views on,
64–65, 67, 151
purification of, 94, 113, 115, 139, 165
three primary, 46, 66–67, 78, 80
(*see also* ida nadi; pingala nadi;
sushumna nadi)
enlightened beings (*karma
sannyasis*), 133
Essence of Yoga, The (Feuerstein), 98

Facets of Indian Thought
(Heimann), 1
fair witness, 100

Jnana Yoga, 23–24
Joubert, Joseph, 67
joy, as obstacle, 127

kaivalya (aloneness, isolation), 100,
    112, 182
Kaivalyadhama, 113
kaleidoscopes, 26–27
Kali Yuga, 42, 43, 44, 132, 152
Kama, 46–47, 113
Kanphata yogis, 140
Kapstein, Matthew, 140–41
karma, 19
    defining, 132
    and dharma, relationship
        between, 131
    reincarnation and, 134, 135
    three ripenings (trivipaka), 134–35
    three states of, 133, 134
    types of, 132–33
Karma and Creativity (Chapple), 135
Karma Yoga, 149
Kashmir Shaivism, 31
Katha Upanishad, 19, 72, 73
Kaula Jnana Nirnaya, 55, 70
kha (zero), 4–5, 7
Kimpurushas, 35
kleshas, 55, 120–22, 179
knots (granthi), 72–73. See also three
    knots (tri granthi)
knowledge
    correct, eight ways to obtain, 106
    as limitation, 54
    wrong, 124
Koelman, G. M., 179
Kramrisch, Stella, 50
Krishna, 123–24
Krishna, Gopi, 111

Krishnamurti, Jiddu, 29, 33, 87, 100
Krita Yuga, 42, 43, 44
Kriya Yoga, 99
Kshemaraja, 35
Kularnava Tantra, 87–88,
    89–90, 157
kundalini, 65, 75, 145, 146
Kundalini (goddess), 111
kundalini shakti, 56–57
Kundalini Yoga, 84
Kung bushmen, 66

Laghu Avadhuta Upanishad, 105
Lakshmi, 58
language, investigating, 7
Larson, Gerald, 28, 81, 178
Laws of Manu, 88
Laya Yoga, 82
liberation (moksha), 19
    bodiless, 152, 182
    desire for (mumukshu), 23–24,
        63, 180
    eight methods, 106
    fast and slow tracks, 29–30
    on palm of hand, 174
    in Patanjali Yoga, 28, 29, 181–83
    time in reaching, 81–82, 83
    two paths, 101
    variant views on, 181–83
    in Vedanta, 23
    while living (jivan mukti), 32,
        182, 183
life force, 66, 68, 85
life spans, 32, 43, 144
Light on Pranayama (Iyengar), 147
Light on Yoga (Iyengar), 140, 145
Lion Pose, 139
Lokaloka Mountains, 35

Myths and Symbols in Indian Art and Civilization (Zimmer), 169

Nada Yoga, 92–93
Nadi Vishvodara, 67
Narada, 73
necessity (*niyati*), 55
neti neti, 13–14, 29
Nirvanam, 1
niyamas (observances), 105, 108–9
   in Hatha Yoga, 72, 103
   in modern practice, 111
   japa as, 158
   lists of, 109
   numbers of, 70, 102, 104, 107, 149
   in Patanjali Yoga, 60, 102, 117, 122
   special powers and, 175
nonattachment, 97, 100
nonharming (*ahimsa*), 175
nonrecognition, 106–7
nonstop discrimination, 23
numbers
   non-literal, 137–38
   and numerals, difference
     between, xv
   purpose of inventing, 2
   sacred, 50, 98, 140–41, 150–54, 153
   systems without zero, 2–3
   uses of, xiii, 2
   zero as, views on, 3

obstacles
   defining, 122
   "grumpy yogi," 127
   lists of, 123–24
   Patanjali's nine, 124–25, 128
   Sanskrit words for, 123
   six, 71

Olivelle, Patrick, 97
OM, 53, 150
   in breathing practices, 147
   chanting, 93, 106, 161
   as ekakshara, 21
   three syllables of, 167–69
oral tradition, 17, 171
Order of 10 Names, 110
Organ, Troy Wilson, 6

Pada, Gauda, 20
Pancadashi, 12, 63
Panda, N. C., 68
Paramarthasara (Abhinavagupta),
   152
Pashupata Yoga (aka Maheshvara
   Yoga), 102–3
passive witness (*sakshin*), 11
Patanjali, 23–24, 27, 119. See also *Yoga
   Sutra*
Patanjali Yoga, 99
   abhayasa and vairagya in, 100–101
   dualism of, 24, 25–26, 27, 28, 31,
     37–39
   fives in, 60
   and Hatha Yoga, differences
     between, 32, 111
   kleshas in, 55, 120–22
   liberation in, 28, 29, 181–83
   as medical diagnosis and
     treatment, 45
   pairs of opposites in, 28
   pratyahara in, 148
   sun and moon in, 84
   supernatural powers in, 175
path of turning back, 136
path of turning toward the world
   (*pravritti*), 136

serpent, coiled, 74–75. *See also* kundalini

Serpent Power (Avalon), 75

seven deadly sins, 125–26

seven-stage practice, 96–98, 102, 104, 107

Shaivism, 11, 50, 52

Shaivism and the Phallic World (Bhattacharya), 141

Shakti, 46
  fivefold aspect, 55, 56–57
  in Hatha origin story, 82–83
  japa recitation and, 160, 161
  two meanings of, 55

Shakti and Shakta (Avalon), 64

Shakuntala (Kalidasa), 137

Shandilya Upanishad, 107–8, 114, 136

Shankara, 11, 62, 63, 110

Shiva, 11, 32, 86, 158
  asana teachings of, 22, 138
  eight-formed, 137
  five as sacred number of, 50–51
  five cloaks of, 54–55
  in Hatha origin story, 82–83
  in Kashmir Shaivism, 31
  lineage of, 89, 141
  names of, 22
  salutations to, 90
  and Shakti, relationship between, 55, 56–57
  symbols of, 49, 52
  third eye of, 46, 47–49
  world as body of, 35
  See also Rudra (Shiva)

Shiva Nataraj, 53–54, 150

Shiva Samhita, 81, 83, 115, 160

Shiva-Shakti, 46, 49, 56, 183

Shodashi, 164, 167

Shoulder Stand, 144, 145

shruti and smriti, difference between, 171

Shuka (fast path), 29

shunya, 4, 6, 7, 9

Siddha Siddhanta Paddati (Gorakshanath), 36, 55, 56, 70, 159, 160, 180

six cleansing acts (*shat karma*), 111–13

six demonic qualities, 72

six fulfillments, 23

six senses, 62

six waves (*shad urmayah*), 71

six-limb schools, 102, 103–4, 107

16-limbed practices, 107, 161–63

sorrow (*dukha*), 4–5, 19, 63, 71, 73, 108, 125, 126, 173

sound, yogic science of, 155–57

space, 55, 141

speech, tangible, 156–57

Spectrum of Consciousness, The (Wilber), 61–62

stories
  Bahva Teaches Vashkali about Brahman, 7–8
  Bird and the Ant, The, 29–30
  Game of Dice and Naming the Four Yugas, 41–42
  Kitten and the Monkey, The, 101
  Origin of Hatha Yoga, 82–83
  She Who Flows, 77

students
  acceptance as, 89–91, 173
  four levels of, 81–82, 83
  three types, 24

Woods, James, 99, 120
Works and Days (Hesiod), 39, 40

"X + 1 syndrome," 97

Yama, 141
yamas (restraints), 105,
    107–8
    in Hatha Yoga, 72, 103
    in modern practice, 111
    lists of, 109
    numbers of, 70, 104,
        107, 148
    in Patanjali Yoga, 60, 102, 109,
        117, 122
    special powers and, 175
Yamuna River, 76, 78
Yatindra Mata Dipika, 180
yoga
    always changing, 93, 94
    complexity in, 157–58
    first revolution in, 18
    focus of, 52
    four stages of, 91, 92–93
    goal of, 91–92, 95
    gurus in, 86
    in *Katha Upanishad*, 19
    modernization in, 69–70, 122, 138,
        139–40, 145
    multiple systems of, 70
    Northern and Southern schools
        of, 101
    oneness in, 21
    ordered lists in, 117
    Patanjali's use of term, 28
    sessions, time and number of,
        114–16
    two poles of, 98–101

Yoga by the Numbers
    numbers included in, xiii–xv
    Sanskrit conventions used in,
        xv–xviii
Yoga Cudamani Upanishad,
    64, 104
Yoga Nidra (Yoga Sleep), 130
yoga of the pot, 111, 145–46
Yoga Shikha Upanishad, 79, 83–84,
    86, 156–57
Yoga Sutra, 70, 148
    on abhyasa and vairagya, 98–99
    on eight limbs, 102, 103
    on five stages of consciousness,
        117–19
    four chapters in, 45
    on gunas, 36
    on kleshas, 120–22
    nine obstacles in, 123,
        124–25, 128
    supernatural powers in, 174,
        175–80
    yama and niyama in, 107
    See also Vyasa (*Yoga Sutra*
        commentator)
Yoga Tattva Upanishad, 167
Yoga Upanishads, 10, 123, 174
Yoga Yajnavalkya, 67, 158
Yogaraja, 152
You are the World (Krishnamurti), 33

zero, xiii
    impact of, 5–6
    Indian understanding of, 6, 9
    invention of, xiv, 1, 3–4, 5
    nirguna and, 10
    source of word, 7
Zimmer, Heinrich, 8, 90, 169

About the Author

RICHARD ROSEN began his study of yoga in 1980 and took his teacher training at the B.K.S. Iyengar Yoga Institute between 1982 and 1985. In 1987 he cofounded the Piedmont Yoga Studio in Oakland, CA, a school that had a successful run for more than twenty-five years. At various times he served as a contributing editor at *Yoga Journal* and a board member for the California Yoga Teachers Association and the Yoga Dana Foundation. Richard lives in a cottage built in 1906 in beautiful Berkeley, CA.